Understanding Nonverbal Learning Disability

This essential book offers an accessible, evidence-based guide to Nonverbal Learning Disability (NVLD) informed by the most current research, and clinical and educational practice. It provides a thorough explanation of the science behind the condition, alongside ideas, support, and practical tips for managing the everyday challenges of the disorder at school and in family life.

Mammarella, Cardillo, and Broitman describe the main characteristics of the condition from both theoretical and practical points of view, as well as examining the similarities and differences between NVLD and other neurodevelopmental disorders. They explore the cognitive and academic weaknesses and strengths of children with NVLD, and the emotional and social difficulties they may experience. The book also provides a systematic review of scientific studies in this field whilst focusing on issues of diagnostic criteria, as well as assessment and intervention strategies. Practical examples are given for teachers and parents to help support children with NVLD in improving their visuospatial and motor skills, as well as peer-social relations, and in promoting the child's individual abilities.

Understanding Nonverbal Learning Disability is essential reading for parents and practitioners in clinical and educational psychology, and health and social care, and students in these fields.

Irene C. Mammarella is Associate Professor at the Department of Developmental and Social Psychology at the University of Padova, Italy.

Ramona Cardillo is Postdoctoral Fellow at the Department of Developmental and Social Psychology at the University of Padova, Italy.

Jessica Broitman is a psychoanalyst in private practice in Berkeley, California, United States.

Understanding Atypical Development

Series editor: Alessandro Antonietti,
Università Cattolica del Sacro Cuore, Italy.

This volume is one of a rapidly developing series in *Understanding Atypical Development*, published by Routledge. This book series is a set of basic, concise guides on various developmental disorders or issues of atypical development. The books are aimed at parents, but also professionals in health, education, social care and related fields, and are focused on providing insights into the aspects of the condition that can be troubling to children, and what can be done about it. Each volume is grounded in scientific theory but with an accessible writing style, making them ideal for a wide variety of audiences.

Each volume in the series is published in hardback, paperback and eBook formats. More information about the series is available on the official website at: https://www.routledge.com/Understanding-Atypical-Development/book-series/UATYPDEV, including details of all the titles published to date.

Published Titles

Understanding Tourette Syndrome
By Carlotta Zanaboni Dina and Mauro Porta

Understanding Rett Syndrome
By Rosa Angela Fabio, Tindara Caprì and Gabriella Martino

Understanding Conduct Disorder and Oppositional-Defiant Disorder
Laura Vanzin & Valentina Mauri

Understanding Giftedness
Maria Assunta Zanetti, Gianluca Gualdi and Michael Cascianelli

Understanding Nonverbal Learning Disability: A Guide to Symptoms, Management, and Treatment
Irene C. Mammarella, Ramona Cardillo and Jessica Broitman

Understanding Nonverbal Learning Disability

A Guide to Symptoms, Management, and Treatment

Irene C. Mammarella,
Ramona Cardillo, and
Jessica Broitman

Routledge
Taylor & Francis Group
LONDON AND NEW YORK

First published 2021
by Routledge
2 Park Square, Milton Park, Abingdon, Oxon OX14 4RN

and by Routledge
605 Third Avenue, New York, NY 10158

Routledge is an imprint of the Taylor & Francis Group, an informa business

British Library Cataloguing-in-Publication Data
A catalogue record for this book is available from the British Library

Library of Congress Cataloging-in-Publication Data
A catalog record has been requested for this book

ISBN: 978-0-3670-2560-1 (hbk)
ISBN: 978-0-3670-2561-8 (pbk)
ISBN: 978-0-4293-9900-8 (ebk)

Typeset in Sabon
by Deanta Global Publishing Services, Chennai, India

Contents

Authors

Irene C. Mammarella is associate professor at the University of Padova, Italy. Her research interests include neurodevelopmental disorders, such as nonverbal learning disability, specific learning disorders, and autism spectrum disorders. She is the co-founder of a university clinical center for neurodevelopmental disorders (Lab.D.A. srl).

Ramona Cardillo is a postdoctoral fellow at the Department of Developmental and Social Psychology at the University of Padova, Italy. She has carried out research on neurodevelopmental disorders and neuropsychological profiles, especially with regard to autism spectrum disorders without intellectual disability, nonverbal learning disability, and attention-deficit hyperactivity disorder.

Jessica Broitman is a psychoanalyst in private practice in Berkeley, California since 1980 and the co-author of many books and articles on nonverbal learning disability. She is currently involved in several research projects concerning the treatment and understanding of nonverbal learning disability and has a special interest in helping professionals and families understand and treat this disorder.

Preface

Statistical data support the notion that the incidence of developmental disorders, and more generally the presence of atypical behaviors in childhood and youth, is increasing in the population around the world. This does not necessarily depend on the fact that pathological conditions are wide spreading: it might be the outcome of increased interest toward the conditions of children and adolescents, greater diffusion of knowledge about the features of atypical development, or higher levels of sophistication and implementation the diagnostic procedures have reached. In any case, adults who have to accompany and drive the growth of the young generations are challenged to find effective ways to manage situations which require peculiar attention. Specialists who take care of children and adolescents with special needs can do a part of this work. But another part is in charge of people who live with those children and adolescents and interact with them outside the therapeutic setting. The contribution of parents, teachers, and trainers in extra-school domains (such as sport, art, hobbies, edutainment, religious education, social activities) can be relevant. But those people should be knowledgeable about the proper way of communicating, engaging, instructing, monitoring, and tutoring atypically developing children and adolescents in order to support their growth efficiently. This book series tries to fit this need.

The series aims to be a set of basic, concise guides on various developmental disorders or issues of atypical development. The books be focused on providing insights into the aspects of the condition that can be troubling to children and adolescents and what can be done about it. Each volume follows a basic structure and is grounded in scientific theory but written very accessibly for the target audience. Typically, each book faces the following issues:

- Signs and symptoms of the disorder
- What causes the disorder
- Available treatments and therapies
- Living with the condition produced by the disorder
- Practical ways to help children with the disorder and to support caregivers
- Communicating the diagnosis to peers
- Cultural differences and sensitivities.

Books include the description of some case-studies, practical examples, and tasks and exercises to be proposed to children and adolescents, as well as check-lists and suggestions to improve the quality of life of children and their family, to support school achievement, and to enhance adaptation and inclusion in social life.

The series is addressed to parents, caregivers, and professionals, with particular emphasis on health, social care, and education. The books are of value to practitioners in clinical and educational psychology, counselling, mental health, nursing, teacher training, child welfare, social work and youth work as well. Professionals and trainees involved in relevant medical disciplines - including midwives, health visitors, school nursing, and public health professionals - and those in general practice, as well as those involved in education, including teachers, classroom assistants, and all those concerned with Early Years, can benefit from the books.

Alessandro Antonietti
Department of Psychology – Catholic University of the Sacred Heart, Milan, Italy
Editor of the series *Understanding Atypical Development*

Introduction

Nonverbal learning disorder (NVLD) has been written about and discussed for the roughly 60 years since it was named and described by Johnson and Mykelbust (1967). Recent work shows that 3 to 4 percent of the population of children in the United States are likely to have NVLD (Margolis et al., 2020). Interest in understanding and studying NVLD has grown significantly over the last 20 years, and several books and publications have recently been written (Cornoldi, 2016; Broitman et al., 2020; Davis & Broitman, 2011, 2013, 2006, 2007; Palombo, 2006; Tanguay, 2002). Few of these were targeted directly to parents and educators, and none were written by researchers or experts in the field (e.g., Burger, 2004; Tanguay, 2000; Tanguay, 2001). Those books are, of course, useful, since they offer the viewpoint of parents living in similar situations. However, as every child with or without NVLD is unique, children suffering from the same condition may or may not have similar symptoms, and each has differing circumstances. Unlike many other neurodevelopmental disorders, this is not a well-known disorder, and there are few sources of information on the best practices and types of support offered at schools or for everyday situations, so the parents of children with NVLD have fewer resources at hand. This book adds to the previous body of knowledge as a useful and unique resource specifically for parents and teachers offering a broader and up-to-date vision of our current understanding of NVLD.

We begin our book with a systematic review of the scientific studies in this field, adding practical guidelines for intervention for both parents and teachers based on information from research and from clinical and educational practice. We describe the condition of NVLD from both theoretical and practical points of view, seeking to bring together the most recent results from research with the most important knowledge from clinical and educational practice. This is in order to support parents and teachers to help NVLD children to best achieve their potential by benefiting from tailored intervention at home, in the classroom, and in social contexts. To illustrate these concepts, practical examples drawn from clinical cases are presented that accompany the reader throughout the book.

In the first chapter, we offer a clear description of the main characteristics of the disorder, including the cognitive and academic weaknesses and strengths of children with NVLD and their emotional and social difficulties. Updated information about the definition of this condition, based on the results of the consensus conference held at Columbia University Irving Medical Center (CUIMC) and sponsored by The NVLD Project, in which two authors of this book were involved (ICM and JB), are included in the first chapter.

In the second chapter, we present a systematic overview of the literature from past theoretical models to the present research and diagnostic criteria. The issue of assessment and the intervention strategies are addressed, and general guidelines for teachers and parents are reported. In order to help the reader in understanding the meaning of the research findings and technical terms, we have added boxes explaining the scientific findings and the specific terms cited in this chapter. The similarities and differences between the NLD condition and other neurodevelopmental disorders are explained in Chapter 3. This chapter ends with a discussion about overlap among disorders and the importance of considering the development of symptoms over the life course. In the fourth chapter, tips for teachers dealing with the academic difficulties of children with NVLD are provided. We added practical examples and activities which could be useful for managing children with NVLD in the school context. Finally, in the last chapter, the parents' roles are considered, and again, we suggest practical tips for providing support for the everyday challenges of the disorder. Suggestions for improving visuospatial and motor skills as well as peer-social relations, are addressed and recommendations about different intervention methods to compensate for the weaknesses and promote the abilities of the child are given.

We hope that in writing this book, we are sharing the best practices for optimizing the development of children with NVLD and helping teachers and parents provide the best aid, specifically tailored for the characteristics of each child.

Chapter 1

What Is Developmental Visuospatial Disorder (or Nonverbal Learning Disability)?

Signs and Symptoms

1.1 Nonverbal Learning Disability (Developmental Visuospatial Disorder)

We begin with a description of the main characteristics of nonverbal learning disability (NVLD) through the depiction of two Italian children, Fabrizio and Alex (names and identifying details changed to protect their privacy), throughout this chapter, and we will follow them in other chapters of this book.

Fabrizio is a brown-haired, 9-year-old child. He has a good vocabulary, and he likes to read children's books and watch scientific documentaries (mainly regarding animals) on TV. During the first years of primary school, he encountered some problems with his handwriting skills. He wrote slowly, the shape of his letters was irregular, and he was not able to keep them correctly aligned on the page. His parents also reported that Fabrizio was confused by new places and encountered difficulties when orienting himself in new environments. In light of these difficulties, his school teachers suggested to Fabrizio's parents that he have a neuropsychological evaluation. Initially, he was referred to a specialized clinical developmental center when he was 7 years old. At that time, the staff immediately noticed his visuospatial processing difficulties with copying complex figures and in fine-motor skills (i.e., grasping small objects and fastening clothing). However, his gross-motor abilities, including walking, running, sitting, and other activities, were in line with other children of the same age. He also showed some difficulties in interacting with peers; he was described as sensitive and insecure, without confidence when playing with peers, and uncomfortable and concerned about his performance due to his visuospatial and fine-motor difficulties.

Alex is a 14-year-old eighth grader who seems older than his age and is passionate about rowing. He loves learning new languages and hates mathematics. Alex likes to talk and describes his thoughts in detail. He is well aware of his weaknesses, naming them as drawing, mathematics, interpreting graphs and diagrams, and fine-motor skills. He was referred for a neurodevelopmental assessment because of his difficulties with school achievement, which were described as slow, labored penmanship, difficulties in solving advanced mathematical problems, and difficulties in recognizing geometric concepts and figures. In fact, during the neuropsychological assessment, his performance was poor in all these domains. Unlike most of his peers, he does not like video games or using social media but prefers to talk with "real" people. In addition, he sometimes appears lost in his own thoughts. Both Fabrizio and Alex received a diagnosis of NVLD. Although there are age differences between the two children, it is clear from these brief descriptions that they share some characteristics: good verbal and language skills, and poor visuospatial processing and fine-motor abilities. We suggest that these are, in fact, the main characteristics of children with NVLD. However, as you will see, we believe that the characteristics of NVLD are quite varied and more nuanced, and we intend to explain the reasons why. We do, however, see a consistent pattern of strengths and challenges. Assets of children with NVLD often include early speech and vocabulary development, a relative strength in auditory/verbal rote memory, often early reading skills, and excellent spelling skills. Difficulties usually include problems in visual–spatial processing (the main deficit), organizational/executive function challenges, academic struggles (typically math), social functioning, and fine-motor coordination issues. Associated difficulties could include psychological issues, specifically during adolescence (Cornoldi, Mammarella & Fine, 2016).

Although many experts and practitioners, working around the world, frequently encounter children with characteristics similar to those described in Fabrizio and Alex, they often fail to use the diagnostic label of NVLD. A recent study by Margolis et al. (2020), for example, found that 3–4 percent of the population of children in the United States are likely to have NVLD. We hypothesize that one possible reason why NVLD is undiagnosed might be because it is not yet fully recognized by the scientific community. In several scientific publications (Broitman et al., 2020; Cornoldi, Mammarella, & Fine, 2016; Mammarella, & Cornoldi, 2019), we explained that this disorder is still not listed in the international diagnostic manuals (such as the Diagnostic and Statistical Manual of Mental Disorders [DSM 5]; APA, 2013). Briefly, the history of NVLD is quite recent. Dyslexia, for example, was described for the first time in 1881. However, the concept of a nonverbal learning disability only dates back to 1967, when Johnson and Myklebust (1967) in their insightful work presented a description of children with an average verbal intelligence who had difficulties in the nonverbal aspects of their environment.

Moreover, it is worth noting that a nonverbal learning disability is a complex disorder. From the beginning, the description of these children suggested the presence of mainly visuospatial processing deficits, but some of their other symptoms resembled different clinical profiles such as autism spectrum disorder, developmental coordination disorder, specific learning disorders, or attention-deficit hyperactivity disorder (ADHD), making their diagnosis challenging (Broitman et al., 2020; Cornoldi, Mammarella, & Fine, 2016). In 2011, Spreen strongly criticized the validity of the nonverbal learning disability diagnosis and concluded that there was little evidence to support its use in clinical practice. In particular, he observed that contrary to expectations, it seems that this disorder occurs only quite rarely, and he disapproved the inclusion of socioemotional symptoms as a core symptom of this profile.

It is worth noting that it is currently acceptable to describe complex clinical profiles with various symptoms involving different neuropsychological domains. Now, both researchers and clinicians agree on the existence of a dimensional approach (DSM-5; APA, 2013), which considers the functioning of a given individual along different dimensions. For example, the idea that children with ADHD, mainly showing attention and hyperactivity deficits, often present socioemotional difficulties is broadly accepted (Hodgens, Cole, & Boldizar, 2000; Hoza et al., 2005; Mrug, Hoza, Pelham, Gnagy, & Greiner, 2007). Peer and teacher reports reveal that children with ADHD like other children more than they are liked (Hoza et al., 2005; Capodieci, Crisci, & Mammarella, 2019) and have fewer friends, appear lonelier, and engage in fewer activities relative to their typically developing peers (Heiman, 2005). In addition, children with autism spectrum disorders often show attention (Murray, 2010; Bühler, Bachmann, Goyert, Heinzel-Gutenbrunner, & Kamp-Becker, 2011) or motor coordination problems (see, for a meta-analysis, Fournier, Hass, Naik, Lodha, & Cauraugh, 2010).

However, while comorbidity is now well accepted, it still remains a significant problem in the field inhibiting the use of the diagnosis of a nonverbal learning disability, as there are currently no "official" shared diagnostic criteria for this disorder. Trying to move a step forward toward finding a consensus on the inclusion and exclusion criteria for nonverbal learning disability, based on a systematic review of the literature, Cornoldi, Mammarella, and Fine (2016) suggested some criteria for its diagnosis.

In May 2017, a conference was held at Columbia University Irving Medical Center (CUIMC). This conference, sponsored by The NVLD Project, was led by Dr. Prudence Fisher and hosted at CUIMC. The consensus group included NVLD global experts, such as Drs. Jessica Broitman, Joseph Casey, John (Jack) M. Davis, Jodene Fine, Irene C. Mammarella, Amy Margolis, Doug Riis, and Margaret Semrud-Clikeman. The scientific advisors to the consortium included Drs. Geraldine Dawson, Michael Furst, Stephen Hinshaw, James McCracken, Mark Riddle, Peter Satzmari, Benedetto Vitiello, and Agnes Whitaker. They were joined by educators from Mary McDowell School and Winston Preparatory School in NYC, which offer programming for students with NVLD, and policy makers from the National Center for Learning Disabilities (NCLD).

Members of The NVLD Project's Board of Directors and Advisory Board also attended these meetings, and all together, they formed a consensus work group. The group's objective was to find a consensus definition of nonverbal learning disability and to have this diagnosis included in future editions of the international diagnostic manuals. Additionally, the conference focused on generating a name for NVLD that would be descriptive and would delineate NVLD based on its defining deficits rather than a description focusing on what it is not (nonverbal). The consensus group arrived at the name *developmental visual–spatial disorder* and generated a definition written within the style of *Diagnostic and Statistical Manual 5* (DSM5) diagnostic criteria. In contrast to previous research definitions, wherein criteria are defined by the neuropsychological test profile, the clinical definition is based largely on behavioral features. Like several other neurodevelopmental disorders in DSM5 (language disorder, specific learning disorder, and intellectual disability), NVLD does require some psychological testing to make a diagnosis (Broitman et al., 2020).

The attendees agreed to change the name from *nonverbal learning disability* to *developmental visuospatial disorder* (DVSD) to reflect that visuospatial processing difficulty is what differentiates these children from others and to disconnect it from the term *nonverbal*, which is confusing, as the label usually reveals the nature, rather than the absence, of the problem (Cornoldi et al., 2016). Another reason for changing the name was that also the term *learning disability* is misleading. It is true that some symptoms concern academic achievement (i.e., mathematical skills and reading comprehension), but children with nonverbal learning disability may have academic weaknesses that are not always associated with dramatically poor school results (see Cornoldi et al., 2016). Moreover, they may fail in academic areas as a consequence of their weaknesses in visuospatial processing.

The group defined a set of behavioral criteria for NVLD that could be submitted to the *Diagnostic and Statistical Manual 5* (DSM5) for consideration of NVLD as a distinct disorder.

As stated in Broitman et al. (2020), inclusion of NVLD in the DSM5 could potentially improve a number of things for individuals with NVLD. Inclusion in DSM would provide improved identification of individuals with NVLD and thus, communication among treating professionals. Inclusion would also provide access to care by allowing billing for treatment. Currently, individuals with NVLD tend to receive diagnoses that capture some of their functional impairments but do not signal the hallmark feature of NVLD, a visual–spatial deficit. *The International Statistical Classification of Diseases and Related Health Problems, Tenth Revision* (ICD-10) provides a code for individuals with visuospatial deficit (R41.842), which may capture NVLD. Finally, inclusion in DSM5 would encourage and support research on treatment by providing a clear set of diagnostic criteria (Broitman et al., 2020).

As defined by the consensus group, the main (A) criteria for developmental visual–spatial disorder (formerly NVLD) specify seven dimensions of visual–spatial processing in which an individual may have difficulties. In order to meet the criteria for the disorder, an individual must have problems in four of seven areas. One strength of the definition is the careful delineation of these seven aspects of visual–spatial processing. As reported in Broitman et al. (2020), there are a few extant studies showing that relative to individuals with ASD or ADHD, children with NVLD have deficits in visual–spatial construction or processing (Mammarella, Cardillo, & Zoccante, 2019; Semrud-Clikeman, Walkowiak, Wilkinson, & Christopher, 2010). However, to date, there is no comprehensive study looking systematically at low-level visual and higher-order visual–spatial processing in children with NVLD. The A criteria specified in the new definition will now provide an important set of testable criteria.

The main (A) criteria are described as persistent deficits in processing and integrating visual and spatial information. The criteria are to be met based on a clinical synthesis of the individual's history (developmental, medical, family, and educational school reports) and psychoeducational or neuropsychological assessment. Moreover, for a diagnosis, the individual must have an impairment in some life activity in addition to meeting the A criteria. The following are the seven areas:

1. Visuospatial awareness (e.g., awareness of own body in space or personal space of others, orienting to new environments)
2. Visuospatial construction (e.g., copying visually presented material, planning, orienting, or organizing stimuli that are visual–spatial in nature, drawing, assembling objects)
3. Visuospatial memory (e.g., remembering patterns and designs, recalling layout of environments, holding spatial information in mind while simultaneously acting on that information)
4. Visuospatial scanning/tracking (e.g., finding information on a page/poster/screen, etc. when there are a lot of distracting images or text, locating things in the presence of clutter, maneuvering in places or situations where other people or things are moving around quickly and in different directions)
5. Spatial estimation (e.g., judging distance, quantity, or time, appropriately using the space on a page, allowing enough time to cross a street when traffic is coming)
6. Three-dimensional thinking (e.g., imagining how things will look when rotated, route finding, following directions to a location)
7. Interpreting information presented pictorially (e.g., diagrams, maps, figures, graphs, analog clocks)

As reported in Broitman et al., 2020, by framing DVSD as a single deficit disorder, the consensus group sought to emphasize the importance of the visual–spatial deficit as the hallmark defining feature of the disorder. This also distinguishes DVSD from other neurodevelopmental disorders. Thus, including DVSD will allow millions of children to be identified as having a neurodevelopmental disorder that requires intervention. Currently, there are no diagnoses in DSM5 that encompass visual–spatial deficits.

This group of experts continues working on their main objective of including DVSD in the Neurodevelopmental Disorders section of the DSM, currently focusing on identifying and conducting the specific empirical studies that would be needed before a submission could be made to DSM5. Thus, from now, we will use the term DVSD to refer to children with this problem. The exception to this will be in Chapter 2, where we describe previously research focused on NVLD, as it had be called. In the next sections, we will describe the main difficulties and the associated symptoms referred to earlier. Although there are no studies that describe the developmental changes, we will try to highlight what parents and teachers may observe at different ages.

1.2 Visuospatial Processing Difficulties

Visuospatial abilities are important in several everyday activities, influencing academic success in science, technology, engineering, and mathematics (STEM), navigation, wayfinding, and sporting activities (Jansen & Lehmann, 2013; Labate, Pazzaglia, & Hegarty, 2014; Wai, Lubinski, & Benbow, 2009).

In the psychological literature, *visuospatial abilities* is an umbrella term that includes different specific skills, such as visuo-constructive, mental rotation, perspective-taking abilities, and so on.

For example, we refer to visuo-constructive abilities as the skills needed to put parts together to form a single whole (Simic, Khan, & Rovet, 2013). These skills are usually assessed by administering tasks in which participants reconstruct a whole figure from a number of different local parts, as in a puzzle, but copying geometric drawings is also often considered as a visuo-constructive or visuo-motor ability. Most children with DVSD fail in those tasks. In everyday situations, parents may observe whether their child likes playing with puzzles or bricks, drawing, filling shapes by using colors, and so on.

For example. mental rotation, which is a visuospatial skill, is the ability to maintain, manipulate, and rotate a mental image into a different orientation in space (Guillot, Hoyek, & Collet, 2012). This ability is often used in daily life, for example, when people have to solve mathematical problems, and it may also involve the mental rotation of body parts or shapes. A different visuospatial ability strictly related to mental rotation is spatial perspective-taking.

Spatial perspective-taking consists in seeing a space from a different perspective, adopting new imaginary orientations, and mentally viewing a scene from an external viewpoint (Pearson, Ropar, & Hamilton, 2013). This spatial transformation process is particularly important in "large-scale" spatial activities, when individuals can imagine "being part of" or "moving through" a space (Münzer, Fehringer, & Kühl, 2018). In fact, tasks investigating spatial perspective-taking abilities have revealed an important role in predicting people's environment-learning (Allen, Kirasic, Dobson, Long, & Beck, 1996; Pazzaglia & De Beni, 2006), navigating, and wayfinding abilities (Kozhevnikov, Motes, Rasch, & Blajenkova, 2006; Schmidt, Tinti, Fantino, Mammarella, & Cornoldi, 2013).

Mental rotations and perspective-taking tasks are highly involved in many daily activities. Let's think back to every time you have tried to assemble a piece of furniture. In this task, both mental rotation and perspective-taking skills are required. Most children with DVSD fail in these tasks. As previously mentioned, visuospatial skills sustain academic success in science and mathematics (Uttal, Miller, & Newcombe, 2013; Mammarella, Lucangeli, & Cornoldi, 2010), navigation and wayfinding (Labate, Pazzaglia, & Hegarty, 2014; Hegarty, Montello Richardson, Ishikawa, & Lovelace, 2006), and sporting activities (Jansen & Lehmann, 2013). Thus, usually, parents more often pay attention to the consequences of visuospatial difficulties in academic situations (such as mathematics, science, and geometry), or in navigation and wayfinding failures. We will talk about academic strengths and differences in the following sections.

1.3 Children with Developmental Visuospatial Disorder at Different Ages

Currently, there are no longitudinal data on children with DVSD. However, based on previous studies and on our experience with children with this disorder, we will summarize the main changes observed throughout different developmental periods in order to highlight signs that parents and teachers might observe. We caution, however, that with possible challenges in four major areas (executive functions, social, academic, and motor coordination) in conjunction with a spatial deficit, every child with DVSD has a unique profile and will look different. We will use excerpts from

Davis and Broitman (2011) *Nonverbal learning disabilities in children* to share common developmental markers.

1.3.1 Early Signs of Visuospatial Difficulties

As one of the authors (JB) has previously published in Broitman et al. (2020), Davis and Broitman (2011), and Broitman and Davis (2013), we have known since Piaget (Inhelder & Piaget, 1964), that in the first stage of development (i.e., the sensorimotor stage, in the first 2 years of development), much learning is about the child's interactions with his or her environment on a sensory and/or perceptual level.

The "typical" amount of exposure to sensorimotor learning, however, tends to be less for the infant, toddler, and preschooler with DVSD (Davis & Broitman, 2011). As Rourke (1995) noted in describing children with this disorder, "these children remain essentially sedentary, exploring the world not through vision or locomotion, but rather through receiving verbal answers to questions posed about the immediate environment" (p. 8). The disparity between early language development, especially vocabulary, and the delays in motor development in the child is most notable in the early years. Anecdotal reports from parents of children with DVSD often state that their children would sit and point at an object, saying what they wanted, rather than crawling towards it. In anticipation of normal exploration, one parent spoke of how she baby-proofed her house to protect her child, yet her child never crawled to or tried to open anything (Davis & Broitman, 2011). Many of these children do not use typical toddler toys or enjoy coloring or drawing. They usually lack interest in putting puzzles together or are unable to do so (Johnson, 1987). Returning to one of the children we introduced at the beginning of this chapter, Alex's parents informed us that he started talking early (he pronounced his first words at 10 months), and while he easily learned to express his needs, he never played with even the simplest building blocks.

Parents are often confused when their extremely verbal child is not developing consistently across developmental lines. They may have unwarranted and inaccurate expectations based on inappropriate assumptions about their child's superior language development (Broitman et al., 2020; Davis & Broitman, 2011). Problems for the child can become exacerbated when poor motor and spatial development disappoint and confound the parents. Early sensorimotor exploration is important in the child's development, since learning depends upon the interaction of the child with the environment (Piaget, 1972). The brain develops secondary to its interactions with the environment, developing neural networks that then create neural efficiency. Although children with DVSD are interacting with their environment, the interactions are often more verbal and observational and less motor and spatial, which alters the development of the neural network (Broitman et al., 2020). It is likely that less interaction and practice exploring the environment with the body leads to reduced efficiency in motor skills compared with children with many more hours of practice. In turn, as they grow older, children with less confidence in their motor skills may be less inclined to engage in activities that demand them, which further reduces their skill growth and development (Davis & Broitman, 2011).

1.3.2 Early Primary School (Age 5–9)

Kindergarten teachers may notice problems in fine-motor skills that have not been noted earlier in a child with DVSD. Our other Italian child Fabrizio's developmental story may be a useful example of the characteristics of DVSD in this age period. During kindergarten, the child struggled more than peers with items such as scissors, crayons, or pencils, and also, poor inclination to draw or to perform fine-motor activities was observed. In general, in this age period, children with DVSD may also show difficulties in completing puzzles, playing with constructional toys such as Lego, or acquiring complex motor skills such as riding a tricycle or bicycle (Davis & Broitman, 2011). As demands for writing and drawing increase, the teacher may notice motor immaturity in children with DVSD compared with their typically developing peers. The teacher may turn to expert practitioners, or learning specialists as they are referred to in the United States, for consultation and guidance. After observing the child, the practitioner might provide an evaluation or offer specific treatments (we will briefly present a typical assessment of children with DVSD in the next sections). This happened to Fabrizio. In his first years of primary school, Fabrizio encountered problems with his handwriting skills (including incorrect pencil grip, poor handwriting legibility, and difficulties in keeping letters aligned on the page). It was for this reason that Fabrizio's school teachers suggested his parents obtain a neuropsychological evaluation from a specialized clinical developmental center. The clinicians analyzed his performance and observed and diagnosed the visuospatial and fine-motor difficulties.

Sometimes, children with DVSD may be referred for help with nonphonological reading difficulties (Pennington, 1991), but intervention may be premature (Davis & Broitman, 2011). Rourke (1995) noted that despite those difficulties, most will develop basic reading skills without intervention. These children often experience a delay in orthographic processing—the learning and processing of phoneme/grapheme connections such as early alphabet learning—a skill that underlies basic reading. However, since there is a somewhat limited number of letters, the contention is that as these become overlearned, the process becomes less problematic for children.

However, Griffin and Gresham (2002) theorized that reading problems are often associated with difficulties in visual processing, such as tracking. Tracking refers to the ability of the child to stay on the correct line of reading or math without veering off course, which creates confusion and requires extra time for the student to become reoriented. Griffin and Gresham further theorized that these problems are due to visual–spatial processing difficulties and claimed that children with DVSD frequently require tracking training, with as many as 30 percent needing to be retrained in order to read fluently. They suggested that these children obtain a thorough optometric examination that includes an assessment of visual tracking.

Often, children with DVSD develop early math difficulties, although some use their verbal memory strengths to help them compensate through third grade and occasionally beyond (Davis & Broitman, 2011). A difficulty in discriminating or estimating quantity, such as comparison of magnitude, may be present. During primary school, the symptoms are likely to emerge more clearly, with demonstration of both strengths and weaknesses associated with DVSD. Strengths should be observed in verbal activities (e.g., reading decoding and recitation of math facts) and difficulties seen in handwriting, conceptual mathematics, geometry, and math-based science. In any case, as the difficulties presented in mathematics by DVSD children mainly involve the visuospatial aspects of mathematics, the consideration of the overall mathematical performance should be associated with a more analytical and deep consideration of crucial tasks such as written calculation and geometry, in which typical errors can be observed. Children with DVSD are likely to make visuospatial errors in written calculations (i.e., confusing columns, carrying/borrowing errors) and write mirrored numbers (see Osmon, Smerz, Brown, & Plambeck, 2006; Mammarella, Lucangeli, & Cornoldi, 2010). If not earlier, concerns begin to develop during this period about social perception and pragmatic language development. Further, boys and girls with DVSD can present with clinical signs of anxiety, depressive symptoms, attention problems, and low self-esteem (Palombo & Berenberg, 1999; Mammarella et al., 2013).

These children can also begin to have social difficulties. For example, Fabrizio showed some difficulties in interacting with peers and was described by parents and teachers as sensitive and as having a lack of self-confidence when playing with peers. It remains unclear whether these children experience these social problems due to processing issues. For example, social difficulties may result from difficulty in processing facial expressions and social signals as well as reduced executive functioning and novel problem-solving ability (Dimitrovsky, Spector, Levy-Shiff, & Vakil, 1998; Semrud-Clikeman, Fine, & Bledsoe, 2014). They might even result from reduced interaction with peers due to sensorimotor issues (Hale & Fiorello, 2004). Clearly, further research is required to evaluate these hypotheses.

In early elementary school, they are more likely to have been seen for pragmatic language difficulties in social discourse. It is believed to bode well for youngsters if these issues are identified early and intervention begins before the child falls behind, allowing secondary features, especially anxiety, to develop (Palombo & Berenberg, 1999).

Even though children with these processing difficulties may struggle and become frustrated by math and written expression, they tend not to be referred to special educators at this time, because they perform *well enough*. Their superior verbal skills often cause educators and parents to assume that their difficulties arise from insufficient effort or difficulty in paying attention. Rourke (1995) wrote that young children with these symptoms are often misdiagnosed with ADHD. Unfortunately, such misdiagnoses can lead to a host of self-esteem problems and psychological issues, particularly when appropriate interventions are withheld (Cornoldi, Mammarella, & Fine, 2016).

1.3.3 Later Elementary and Middle School (Age 10–13)

As academic subjects become more abstract, and more independent work is expected, children with DVSD often begin to experience greater difficulties (Davis & Broitman, 2011). Executive function problems increase. At the same time, more demands are placed on social skills, creating significant additional stress and frustration that can elevate anxiety and make academic progress difficult. Teachers become alarmed and mention their concerns at parent conferences. Parents ask for help for their children, and public or private school wheels are set in motion (Hale & Fiorello, 2004; Telzrow & Bonar, 2002). Providing the best assistance for the student with DVSD can become problematic because so much depends on who gets involved and what they already know. The child's parents need to educate themselves to become more knowledgeable, as they will need to become increasingly involved in their child's treatment team (Davis & Broitman, 2011).

1.3.4 High School (Age 14–18)

If the child with DVSD has managed to navigate the complex middle school environment fairly successfully, the high school experience becomes the next challenge (Davis & Broitman, 2011). During high school, social skills can become a source of even greater concern, as social stresses such as the demands of dating are increased. Advanced math and sciences will also be more challenging. Alex, for example, showed difficulties in solving advanced mathematical problems and in recognizing geometric concepts and figures. Even with a problem he had seen before, if it was modified slightly, he had trouble recognizing and solving it. Alex also showed problems with interpreting graphs, charts, and maps. In addition, increased demands on executive functioning, such as in written expression and advanced reading skills, can present major challenges. Research is mixed regarding whether students with DVSD are more at risk for psychiatric disorders such as depression, with some studies finding increased levels of depression (Brumback, 1985; Fletcher, 1985; Rourke, Young, & Leenaars, 1989) and others finding no increased risk for psychiatric disorders (Forrest, 2004; Mokros, Poznanski, & Merrick, 1989). It is possible that these contradictory findings are due to the significant differences in age, race, and income among the different studies, or differing definitions for classification of eligibility in a particular study, given the wide range of criteria used in research on DVSD; therefore, further research is needed in order to better understand the psychopathological consequences (Davis & Broitman, 2011).

However, with interventions, accommodations, and modifications, students with DVSD are often able to tap into their skill sets and experience success. It is crucial to understand the strengths and weaknesses of every student, and it is at least equally important that the student's strengths be recognized and enhanced as it is to remediate relative weaknesses or deficits. Positive skill sets might include acquisition of a second language, drama, certain aspects of the arts, language arts, and some of the more language-based sciences.

Transition planning becomes essential at this stage, and decisions about further education need to be made. In our experience, students who have not become too demotivated or demoralized can move on to successful adulthood if they, with the help of their parents and coaches, choose wisely with special regard for their strengths (Davis & Broitman, 2011). Students with DVSD often interact better with adults than with their peers. Personal accounts written by people with DVSD suggest that adulthood may bring more successful interactions and relationships. Overall, early accurate diagnosis and appropriate interventions are crucial to the well-being of the person with NVLD.

1.4 Assessment of Children with Developmental Visuospatial Disorder

Once parents and teachers observe signs of DVSD and the behaviors we have described in the previous sections, they may request a broader assessment to be conducted in order to better understand the strengths and weaknesses of their child. How this process proceeds will depend upon where they are located. In Italy, for example, parents may request a complete neuropsychological assessment by specialized practitioners in both public or private centers specializing in neurodevelopmental disorders. After this evaluation, if the child satisfies the diagnostic criteria for a DVSD diagnosis, he or she is recognized as having special educational needs. Children with special educational needs may have access to all the school measures provided for children with learning disabilities, and schools are required to complete an Individual Educational Plan (IEP) tailored to the specific child's needs.

Similarly, in the United States, every state has its own regulations, but the Individuals with Disabilities Education Act (IDEA) enables all parents to request an IEP meeting with the public schools to try to get additional help for their child, or for young adults to determine eligibility for the Americans with Disabilities Act (ADA). As described in Broitman et al. (2020), the Entitlement Law (IDEA) (which involves the creation of an IEP) states that students with a disability are eligible for a free and appropriate public education (FAPE) if they need special education. The Individualized Education Program (IEP) is an individualized plan, created at an IEP meeting, that establishes the educational goals for eligible students for one school year. In order to begin this process, a parent must request in writing that an IEP meeting be set up. Usually, the learning specialist for the school will facilitate this, but in some instances, the principal will set the ball in motion. If the student is in an American private school setting, or if the family simply prefers this, an assessment might be done privately with a psychologist. In a private practice setting, referrals generally come from a colleague, a parent, a school, or an individual who thinks or has been told that he or she has DVSD. Many services are available to students with disabilities, including:

- Integrated Co-Teaching Class (ICT)
- Speech Therapy (ST)
- Occupational Therapy (OT)
- Transportation
- Assistive technology (AT)
- Push in service
- Pull out service
- Classroom accommodations
- Curriculum modification
- Testing accommodations
- Paraprofessional (crisis, health)
- Bilingual services
- FM unit
- Scribe
- Special Education Teacher Support Services (SETSS)
- Adaptive Physical Education (APE)
- Physical Therapy (PT)

The assessment procedure follows the same phases of the diagnostic process typical of other developmental disorders (i.e., use

Table 1.1 Assessment Areas for Children with DVSD

General areas of the assessment	*Specific areas of the assessment*
General cognitive skills	• Verbal intelligence • Visuospatial intelligence • Fluid reasoning • Quantitative reasoning • Working memory • Processing speed • Total IQ
Attention and executive functions	• Sustained attention (verbal and visual) • Working memory • Inhibition • Shifting
Memory	• Visuospatial working memory • Visuospatial long-term memory
Visuospatial processing	• Visuo-motor and visuo-constructive skills • Spatial mental rotation • Spatial organization and planning
Sensory motor skills	• Fine-motor abilities • Gross-motor abilities • Graphomotor skills
Language—receptive	• Pragmatics and inferences
Academic testing: math	• Math concepts • Math calculation • Math application • Math fluency
Academic testing: written expression	• Handwriting fluency • Spelling • Compositional fluency • Writing mechanics • Composition: narrative and expository
Academic testing: reading	• Reading comprehension • Literal reading • Fluency • Inferential word reading
Affect and behavior	• Depressive symptoms • Anxiety • Social problems • Oppositional • Conduct • Self-esteem

of instruments with recent and valid normative standardization data, and use of multiple informants and sources that test alternate hypotheses) and should include several steps (parent interview, teachers' and parents' report, and an assessment of cognitive and socioemotional skills) in order to arrive at the final diagnosis. For the teachers' report, Cornoldi et al. (2003; the English version is available in Cornoldi et al., 2016) developed the Shortened Visuospatial Questionnaire. This is a checklist for teachers devoted to collecting information about the presence of DVSD symptoms within the classroom environment. The questionnaire includes 18 items and uses a 4-point Likert scale. Ten items concern some of the deficits that, according to previous studies, represent the critical features of DVSD. In particular, items include the child's use of the available space on paper while drawing, visuo-motor coordination, comprehension of visuospatial relations on verbal description, coordination of complex movements, handling of the spatial components of calculation, orientation to space, drawing, visuospatial learning, skills in observing the surrounding environment, and ability to deal with novel objects. There is also a recent version involving self-report for children (Ferrara & Mammarella, 2013; the English version is available in Cornoldi et al., 2016) that captures the awareness of the child of his/her difficulties and can be used to understand how aware of his/her problems the child is.

Different areas should be considered by the practitioner during the assessment procedure. In Table 1.1, we summarize the areas that should be considered for children with DVSD.

Overall, the diagnostic profile is useful not only for planning tailored interventions but also to understand whether the child needs special education services according to the national guidelines of each country. Based on the diagnostic profile, the practitioner can give more specific suggestions to the teachers by considering every subject and by considering the strengths and challenges of the child. To sum up, parents need a thorough evaluation of their child in order to know what their child needs assistance with. When they and/or the team understand this, the actual act of advocacy can begin.

In the next chapters, after an overview of the main research findings, specific suggestions for teachers and parents will be offered.

Chapter 2

Theoretical Models and Research Findings

In this chapter, we will briefly summarize the history of the use of the term nonverbal learning disability. Although in the other chapters we refer to children with this profile with the term developmental visuospatial disorder (DVSD), in the present chapter, we prefer to maintain the original term nonverbal learning disability (NVLD) used in the studies that we have tried to summarize. Given that, in this chapter, we have used many technical terms, to help the reader understand the meaning of the research findings, we have added boxes explaining the specific terms and the test measures used and cited in the text. It is our hope that this information will help explain the difficulty in formalizing the definition, gaining community acceptance, and coordinating research programs.

It is worth noting that compared with other neurodevelopmental disorders, NVLD is a relatively recent term. For example, while Oswald Berkhan offered the description of a child with severe reading difficulties in 1881 in Germany, Sir George Still mentioned attention-deficit hyperactivity disorder (ADHD) in 1902, and Kanner described children with autism spectrum disorder (ASD) in 1943, NVLD emerged only in 1967. This may be in part because the signs of NVLD resemble symptoms of already recognized disorders. Also, researchers and practitioners were not all in agreement that problems with visuospatial processing best differentiated nonverbal learning disability from other disorders.

In addition, for many years, children with low visuospatial skills and average verbal abilities have been called children with "nonverbal learning disability," although the term "nonverbal" is confusing, as it refers to the absence of a verbal problem (Cornoldi et al., 2016). In all other disorders, the name immediately refers to and highlights the main problem of the child. For instance, in specific learning disorders, children show learning difficulties; in ADHD (see Box 2.1), children have attention difficulties and show hyperactivity in their behaviors. In our view, however, it is important for parents and teachers to understand how circuitous the history of the nonverbal learning disability has been and how that has impacted the way in which research studies have progressed. The history of this disorder is a good example of the importance of doing research in the field of developmental disorders and understanding the implications that this research may have on the creation of interventions that can improve the life of children with NVLD.

Box 2.1 Technical Terms Used in This Section and Their Meanings

Technical term	*Meaning*
Attention-deficit hyperactivity disorder (ADHD)	Disorder characterized by inattention, or excessive activity and impulsivity, which are not appropriate for a child's age.
Autism spectrum disorder (ASD)	Disorder that affects communication and behavior, causing significant problems in social interactions. This condition is also characterized by behavioral challenges, including a limited and repetitive pattern of interests and behaviors.
Visuospatial processing	Ability to perceive, analyze, and manipulate visual patterns and images.

2.1 The First Description of Nonverbal Learning Disability

The term "nonverbal learning disabilities" is first attributed to Johnson and Myklebust (1967), who suggested that these children had an average verbal intelligence while showing difficulty in nonverbal aspects of their environment. The typical child was described with "persistent problems in right-left orientation, constructional tasks and arithmetic, whose deficit is not verbal, not academic in the usual sense, but who is unable to comprehend the significance of many aspects of his environment" (1967, p. 272). They defined selective deficits in several areas: the first area of impairment was called visual perception and referred to the ability to encode the whole and the component parts of a configuration and to learn through pictures. Furthermore, these children showed difficulties in processing meaningful gestures and in motor learning, such as handwriting or using objects such as scissors. According to these authors, children with nonverbal learning disability had problems in the visualization of their own body, associated with digital agnosia; other areas of difficulty were spatial orientation, e.g., the ability to establish a spatial relationship of the body with other objects and to recall spatial locations, and left–right orientation. Johnson and Myklebust also associated these dysfunctions with a syndrome described by J. Gerstmann in the first half of the nineteenth century (see Gerstmann, 1940) and characterized by problems in left–right orientation, digital agnosia, dyscalculia, and dysgraphia associated with a left hemisphere parietal dysfunction (see Box 2.2). Moreover, the authors observed two additional nonverbal domains social perception difficulties and problems in the regulation of attention/monitoring systems (Johnson & Myklebust, 1967).

Box 2.2 Technical Terms Used in This Section and Their Meanings

Technical term	*Meaning*
Constructional tasks	Tasks requiring an entire integrated figure to be reconstructed, starting from its single fragments, by drawing or by using three-dimensional objects.
Digital agnosia	Inability to distinguish, name, or recognize the fingers, including the fingers of others, and drawings and other representations of fingers.
Dyscalculia	Condition that affects the ability to perform calculations; it includes a wide range of difficulties with math, such as a deficit in understanding the meaning of numbers and difficulty in applying mathematical principles to solve problems.
Dysgraphia	Disorder of written expression that impairs writing and fine-motor skills.
Left hemisphere parietal dysfunction	Dysfunction that involves the left parietal lobe of the brain.

2.2 The Rourke's "White Matter Model": The Original Conceptualization of NVLD in Previous Research

Rourke (1995) and his colleagues next introduced a developmental neurological approach to studying learning disabilities and proposed the "white matter model" for explaining nonverbal learning disability, which will be described in the following. According to Rourke (1995), this disorder is characterized by deficits grouped into three main areas: neuropsychological, academic, and social-emotional/adaptational. He suggested "a cascade effect" whereby primary neuropsychological deficits lead to secondary deficits, which then lead to tertiary deficits, and so on. Primary neuropsychological deficits include tactile, visual perception, and motor coordination. In turn, secondary deficits (i.e., tactile and visual attention) lead to tertiary deficits, particularly in visuospatial memory, abstract reasoning, and specific aspects of speech and language. Academic deficits involve difficulties with math calculations, mathematical reasoning, reading comprehension, specific aspects of written language, and handwriting. In his model, academic performance, social functioning, and emotional well-being are direct by-products of this constellation of primary, secondary, and tertiary neuropsychological deficits.

Rourke's model has been called the "white matter hypothesis" because according to his view, the nonverbal learning disability syndrome resulted from disturbances in the myelination (white matter) of the extensive fiber tracts that constitute the right hemisphere anatomy. However, he also suggested that the white matter hypothesis could be extended to a wide variety of congenital as well as acquired conditions. Specifically, Rourke proposed that the nonverbal learning disability profile could be found in at least three different situations: 1) children with other diagnoses, such as Asperger syndrome, velocardiofacial syndrome (22q11 deletion), Turner syndrome, agenesis of the corpus callosum, etc., who also have a nonverbal deficit profile; 2) children with a specific nonverbal disorder who do not have severe academic difficulties; and 3) children with a specific nonverbal disorder who also have severe learning problems (see Box 2.3).

It is worth noting, however, that Rourke's model and in consequence, the concept of a nonverbal learning disability were widely criticized by other researchers. In particular, in 2009, Pennington concluded that "we do not have sufficient evidence to accept it as a

Box 2.3 Technical Terms Used in This Section and Their Meanings

Technical term	*Meaning*
Right hemisphere anatomy	The set of structures composing the right half of the brain.
Congenital	A disease or physical abnormality present from birth.
Asperger syndrome	Disorder that is part of the autism spectrum disorders, characterized by significant difficulties in social interaction, restricted and repetitive patterns of behavior and interests, and unimpaired language and intelligence.
Velocardiofacial syndrome (22q11 deletion)	Genetic syndrome defined by the deletion of DNA from chromosome 22 and characterized by heart, craniofacial, behavioral, vascular, central nervous system, and other deficits.
Turner syndrome	Genetic syndrome in which a female is missing (partly or completely) an X chromosome. Common features of the disorder are short stature, ovarian dysfunction, extra folds of skin on the neck, and skeletal and heart abnormalities. Difficulties in processing visuospatial information may be present.
Agenesis of the corpus callosum	Birth defect characterized by a complete or partial absence of the brain structure named the corpus callosum (i.e., the band of white matter connecting the two hemispheres of the brain).
Nonverbal deficit profile	Clinical profile characterized by difficulties with visuospatial skills with possibly associated problems in attention, motor, academic, and social skills.

valid learning disorder apart from either autism spectrum disorder, mathematics disorder or developmental coordination disorder, all of which are covered in the DSM-IV-TR" (p. 248).

Additionally, Spreen (2011) stated that nonverbal learning disabilities were quite rare. Spreen concluded that nonverbal learning disability "remains a hypothesis, but it should not be used in clinical practice unless it is supported by solid research findings" (2011, p. 18).

Other terms have also previously been used to refer to children with a nonverbal learning disability profile, including right hemisphere developmental learning disability (Tranel et al., 1987), visuospatial learning disability (Cornoldi et al., 2003), and deficit in attention, motor control, and perception (Gillberg, Winnegar, & Gillberg, 1993; Gillberg, 2003). Thus, the presence of different labels for a single disorder, in addition to the use of a single term (i.e., nonverbal syndrome) referring to different impairments, gave rise to doubts about the existence of this disorder.

2.3 More Recent Research Findings

Concerns aside, researchers have recently made a remarkable effort to study children who struggle with visuospatial skills with associated potential problems in attention, motor, academic, and social skills but without an associated neurological or genetic syndrome.

Although in past years some critiques were moved regarding NVLD, more recently, a remarkable effort has been made by researchers to define shared criteria for diagnosing these children. This was driven by the need to reach a consistent definition of the profile of this disorder. For this reason, a group of researchers began discussions and planned projects toward the goal of clarifying the definition of NVLD. One of these projects aimed to estimate the prevalence of NVLD in North America (Margolis et al., 2020). This was the first prevalence study of this disorder conducted in a community sample. This is very significant, as all prior studies on the prevalence of NVLD were limited by utilizing a restricted sample (i.e., children with a diagnosis of learning disorder). This study involved three large samples of children who were enrolled in studies centered around brain imaging and the occurrence of psychiatric diagnoses or effects of maternal smoking during pregnancy. The findings suggest that 3–4 percent of children and adolescents in the general population meet the diagnostic criteria for NVLD. This translates to roughly 2 to 3 million children and adolescents in the United States who may have NVLD. Note that they excluded children with potential comorbid ASD in this study because they hoped to estimate the rate of NVLD separately from NVLD that might co-occur with ASD.

In the following section, we will try to summarize more recent studies and to highlight their implications for families and children.

In order to simplify the huge number of studies, we will concentrate those findings in three areas: visuospatial abilities and other neuropsychological functions, academic skills, and social functioning.

2.3.1 *Visuospatial Abilities and Other Neuropsychological Functions*

Although a crucial aspect of the NVLD profile relates to poor visuospatial skills, visuospatial abilities have not been systematically studied (please refer to Box 2.4 for a better definition of the specific terms and tests used in the research studies). We know, for example, that children with NVLD may be impaired in tasks involving visuo-constructive skills that require the reconstruction of fragments belonging to an entire integrated figure by drawing or by using three-dimensional objects (Cornoldi et al., 2016). Some of those tasks require part-to-whole construction, like the Object Assembly subtest of the Wechsler Intelligence Scale for Children (WISC) scale (e.g., Drummond et al., 2005). Previous research revealed that children with NVLD obtained low performances in the Rey–Osterrieth complex figure test (Gross-Tsur et al., 1995; Semrud-Clikeman et al., 2010) and in the Visual-Motor Integration Test (Roman, 1998; Mammarella et al., 2006; Semrud-Clikeman et al., 2010). These tasks require copying by drawing simple or more complex geometrical images (Semrud-Clikeman et al., 2010). Moreover, other research (Cornoldi et al., 1995) suggested that children with NVLD fail in simple tasks requiring the organization of three to four puzzle pieces. Not only visuo-constructive abilities but also visual perception may be impaired. For example, Roman (1998) described a single case of a child with NVLD with specific perceptual difficulty concerning spatial features performing poorly in the Benton Judgment of Line Orientation test (Benton et al., 1983). In this task, children have to find, among a series of lines differently oriented in the space, which one is exactly similar to a target line. Semrud-Clikeman et al. (2010) reported similar findings in a group of children with NVLD compared with Asperger syndrome or ADHD using the same task, and Chow and Skuy (1999) showed that children with NVLD performed less well than children with specific language disorders on gestalt configuration tasks. Finally, Mammarella and Pazzaglia (2010) found that children with NVLD performed worse than controls in visual perception tasks that entailed comparing visual stimuli and locations in space (without involving memory) and in reversing an ambiguous figure.

Another visuospatial skill mainly involved in daily life is visuospatial working memory. This system is responsible for the temporary maintenance and simultaneous processing of visual and spatial information, and it is involved in a large number of everyday tasks, such as map learning and navigation (Denis, Daniel, Fontaine, & Pazzaglia, 2001), and in recalling the positioning of objects in the environment (Zimmer, Speiser, & Seidler, 2003). Mammarella and Cornoldi (2005) and Basso Garcia et al. (2014) observed decreased performance in the backward Corsi blocks task in children with NVLD, which was not present in typically developing children, whereas both typically developing children and those with NVLD had a similar decease in performance with a backward digit span. In addition, poor performances of children with NVLD have been found in several visuospatial working memory tasks requiring them to remember simultaneously or sequentially presented locations (Cornoldi et al., 1999; Mammarella & Cornoldi, 2005a, 2005b). In order to find evidence to distinguish the profiles of children with NVLD and ASD, Mammarella, Cardillo, and Zoccante (2019) compared groups of children with these two disorders with children with typical development in visuo-constructive and visuospatial working memory tasks. They found that the NVLD group's performance was worse in both the visuospatial domains examined (i.e., in visuo-constructive and visuospatial working memory tasks), whereas the group with ASD had a less general difficulty. The authors concluded that the manipulation of visuospatial tasks would enable these two profiles of children to be better distinguished.

Executive functions have been also studied in children with NVLD. In particular, Semrud-Clikeman et al. (2014) collected three measures of executive functioning using the Delis–Kaplan Tests of Executive Functioning (D-KEFS; Delis et al., 2001), finding differences between children with NVLD, children with ASD, and typically developing controls, especially in the trail-making task, which involved visuospatial working memory and sequencing. Overall, these findings support the hypothesis that clinical differences exist between NVLD, ASD, and ADHD. Finally, executive functioning deficits in the Wisconsin Card Sorting Test have also been observed in these children (Fisher, DeLuca, & Rourke, 1997; Semrud-Clikeman et al., 2014). The Wisconsin Card Sorting Test is considered as a measure of cognitive flexibility involving the ability to change the response on the basis of the characteristics of the stimuli (see Box 2.4).

Box 2.4 Technical Terms Used in This Section, Their Meaning, and the Tests Cited in the Text for Measuring Each Skill

Technical term	*Meaning*	*Tests*
Visuo-constructive skills	The ability to reconstruct fragments belonging to an entire integrated figure by drawing or by using three-dimensional objects.	Object assem-blyRey's complex figureVisual-Motor Integration Test
Visual perception skills	The ability to organize and interpret the information that is seen and give it meaning.	Benton Judgment of Line Orientation test
Visuospatial working memory	The ability to temporary maintain while simultaneously processing visual and spatial information.	Corsi blocks task
Executive functions	A set of cognitive processes necessary for the cognitive control of behavior. They are involved in selecting and successfully monitoring behaviors that facilitate the attainment of chosen goals.	Delis–Kaplan TestsWisconsin Card Sorting Test

To summarize, different research has showed that:

- Children with NVLD may present difficulties in different visuospatial tasks involving visuo-constructive, visuo-perceptual, and visuospatial working memory skills.
- Executive dysfunction may emerge in their profile, involving in particular visuospatial working memory, sequencing, and cognitive flexibility.

- Visuospatial skills and executive functions are usually assessed during the diagnostic process. Hence, all this information may aid practitioners to better clarify the profile of strengths and weaknesses of NVLD and to differentiate the clinical profile of children with NVLD from that of other developmental disorders, such as ASD.

In the next chapters, we will better translate how these difficulties may become manifest in everyday life, and how teachers and parents may help children with those problems.

2.3.2 *Academic Performances of Children with NVLD*

It is generally recognized that children with NVLD perform well in reading and poorly in mathematics (e.g., Harnadek & Rourke, 1994; Forrest, 2004). Thus, a series of studies has been carried out to better understand the difficulties of these children in mathematical achievement. For instance, Venneri and co-authors (2003) suggested that the mathematical difficulties of these children may be related to their visuospatial working memory impairments. This hypothesis has been also tested by Mammarella et al. (2010). In their study, the authors found that children with symptoms of NVLD produced more borrowing and carrying errors in written calculation than their peers, and they also found more partial calculation errors and column confusions. In a further study, Mammarella, Bomba, et al. (2013) observed that children with NVLD were impaired in a task requiring them to compare the numerosity of dots, while children with comorbid dyscalculia and dyslexia showed low performance in retrieval of arithmetical facts, which is supported by verbal working memory processes. In addition, some studies examined the SNARC effect (see Box 25), which is interpreted as an automatic association between numbers and space (Hubbard, Piazza, Pinel, & Dehaene, 2005). In a typical SNARC task, generally, participants make faster decisions about small numbers, in terms of reaction times, when stimuli are presented on the left, and faster responses of large numbers when they are presented on the right. In particular, Bachot et al. (2005) found no signs of the typical SNARC effect in children with NVLD compared with typically developing children. The absence of the SNARC effect (see Box 2.5) in a group of children with NVLD has been also replicated by a recent study carried out by Crollen et al (2016). These authors suggested that poor visuospatial skills may

Box 2.5 Technical Terms Used in This Section and Their Meaning

Technical term	*Meaning*	*Tests*
SNARC effect	Automatic association that occurs between the left–right location and the semantic magnitude of a modality-independent number. In the typical SNARC task, when presented with smaller numbers (0 to 4), people tend to respond faster if those stimuli are presented on the left, while when presented with larger numbers (6 to 9), people respond faster if those stimuli are presented on the right.	SNARC task
Mental number line	This refers to a language-independent analogical representation of numerical magnitude in which small numbers are represented on the left and large numbers are represented on the right.	Number-to-position task

produce a basic abnormality in representing numerical magnitudes on an oriented mental number line. In the same study, Crollen et al. (2016) found that the control group outperformed children with NVLD in the number bisection and number comparison tasks, both involving number magnitude but not a physical spatial medium, and in the number-to-position task, which requires both the processing of a number magnitude and the mapping between this magnitude and a spatial medium in the mental number line. Overall, their findings suggest that children with NVLD have less precise numerical representation than typically developing peers. The performance on geometry tasks has been also studied in children with NVLD. Specifically, Mammarella, Giofrè, et al. (2013) showed that children with this disorder perform significantly worse than typically developing children in geometry tasks. Most importantly, the authors observed that a visuospatial working memory deficit explained the difficulty of children with NVLD, but not of typical controls, suggesting that for the NVLD group, the involvement of visuospatial working memory is crucial also in the acquisition of basic intuitive geometrical concepts. Last, Margolis and colleagues have shown that compared with typically developing children, children with NVLD have significant reductions in left hippocampal volume, which was also associated with worse mathematical problem solving (Banker et al., 2020b).

To summarize, overall research studies in the field of mathematics and geometry in children with NVLD seem to suggest that:

- Visuospatial skills are strongly involved in mathematics, for example, in the procedures required to perform written calculations, in understanding fractions and decimal places, and of course, in the mental representation of geometrical figures.
- The difficulties encountered by children with NVLD may be due to their poor visuospatial processing skills. Thus, it is not surprising that children with poor visuospatial abilities underperform peers with typical development in math tasks.

Further studies have examined language and reading comprehension. Although verbal abilities are considered a strength point of the NVLD profile, deficits in the pragmatics of language and, to some extent, in language and reading comprehension have been observed.

The pragmatics of language is the ability to use language effectively and appropriately in interaction with other people and refers to the functional and contextual use of language, including an appreciation of the rules of social discourse, the speaker's purpose in communication, and how language is modified to fit different situations (Tager-Flusberg, 1999). Difficulties in making inferences in language comprehension, particularly with spatial and emotional materials (Worling et al., 1999; Humphries et al., 2004), and impairments in understanding humor have been described (Semrud-Clikeman & Glass, 2008). In another study, Cardillo et al. (2018) found that children with NVLD had a better profile in terms of pragmatics of language than children with dyslexia associated with language impairments. The NVLD group only had difficulties in understanding perceptual metaphoric sentences, opting for literal interpretations. Once again, the presentation of visuospatial material seems to be an important variable to consider for interpreting the performances obtained by the NVLD group.

Moreover, difficulties in understanding spatial descriptions and in developing spatial representations or spatial mental models

(Johnson-Laird, 1983) have been found in children with NVLD. Specifically, children with NVLD had problems in relocating landmarks in a background (Rigoni, Cornoldi, & Alcetti, 1997) and in particular with descriptions in which the overview of the spatial layout is provided without considering the perspective of the individual, but in which cardinal points are used, such as north, south, and so on (Mammarella et al., 2009, 2015). Thus, the studies described here suggest that children with NVLD may show difficulties when they have to both understand and mentally represent visuospatial information, or when language has to be interpreted on the basis of contextual information.

To summarize, the academic performance of children with NVLD may be characterized by good verbal abilities and difficulties in different areas due to their poor visuospatial processing skills, and the potential challenges they may have to deal with are summarized here:

- Poor mathematics skills may result in:
  - Borrowing and carrying errors in written calculation
  - Partial calculation errors and column confusions
  - Difficulties in number comparison tasks and number-to-position tasks
  - Less precise numerical representation than typically developing peers
  - Impairments in geometry tasks
- Difficulties in pragmatics of language may be characterized by:
  - Difficulties in making inferences in language comprehension
  - Impairments in understanding humor
  - Deficit in understanding perceptual metaphoric sentences
- Difficulties in understanding spatial descriptions and in developing spatial representations or spatial mental models may be characterized by:
  - Difficulties in understanding verbal instructions describing how to reach a place
  - Difficulties in representing the shape of a spatial environment (i.e., a park, a building, etc.)

2.3.3 Social Skills in Children with NVLD

With regard to social functioning, some researchers have tested the ability to interpret and recognize facial expressions in children with NVLD (Dimitrovsky et al., 1998; Bloom & Heath, 2010). For example, Bloom and Heath (2010) examined facial affect recognition using a face pool of stimuli of adult faces. Their findings showed that children with general learning disabilities recognized and interpreted facial expressions less accurately than those with NVLD and typically developing adolescents. The authors suggested that it may be the severity, rather than the type, of learning challenge that most influences the ability to interpret facial affects.

Petti et al. (2003) examined basic emotions (happy, sad, anger, fear) in three conditions: faces, gestures (body, no faces), and auditory only. In the auditory only condition, neutral sentences are read using a tone of voice consistent with each of the four emotions. Their results revealed that the NVLD group was less accurate than groups of children with verbal learning disabilities, or typically developing controls, in identifying emotions from body gestures and from adult, but not child, facial emotions. The authors interpreted this finding in terms of the higher familiarity of all groups with children's facial emotions. Additionally, no group differences were found in the interpretation of voices. Thus, this work suggests that children with NVLD might have some weakness in the encoding or interpretation of visual, but not verbal, emotional information. Finally, Semrud-Clikeman et al. (2014) used naturalistic video vignettes of children interacting with one another (CASP; Magill-Evans et al., 1995). Children with NVLD were found to have a similar ability to their typically developing peers to recognize emotions in the actors. In this task, the tone of voice is preserved, but the lexical content is masked. Interestingly, children with NVLD had significantly more difficulty than typical controls in identifying the nonverbal cues, such as facial expression, body language, and prosody. To sum up, in a situation where verbal content is masked and the child must rely on nonverbal information alone in real-time interactions, children with NVLD appeared to understand the interactions but were not able to identify the nonverbal cues as well as typical controls.

NVLD and ASD share some characteristics, such as parent reports of problems in social functioning, even though these difficulties may derive from different underlying deficits. For example, both groups show deficits in social perception, understanding humor, and processing pragmatic language, but some differences in their behavioral presentation must be taken into account (Cardillo, Garcia, Mammarella, & Cornoldi, 2018; Semrud-Clikeman, Fine,

& Bledsoe, 2014; Semrud-Clikeman, Walkowiak, Wilkinson, & Christopher, 2010; Semrud-Clikeman & Glass, 2008). Semrud-Clikeman and colleagues (2013) compared a group of children with NVLD with children with high functioning autism using direct measures of social perception and parent and teacher ratings. Their findings showed that the group with high functioning autism was the most impaired in understanding emotional cues, while both children with NVLD and those with high functioning autism experienced difficulties with nonverbal cues (e.g., difficulties in recognizing the character's emotions from nonverbal cues, like "mouth turned up in a smile" or "eyebrows were raised"). In order to better understand the reactions of children with NVLD to humor, a review was conducted by Semrud-Clikeman and Glass (2008), which considered different studies on autism and NVLD. The authors highlighted that children with autism may have difficulties in understanding jokes and funny stories. Individuals with this diagnosis enjoy humor mostly centered around obsessive topics and not with the intention of sharing humor with others. This kind of humor is described as being of a cognitive nature and being learned rather than for sharing interactions with others. Children with NVLD are reported to have difficulties in understanding humor in part because of a difficulty with understanding multiple meanings of words and a tendency to be literal in conceptualization. Sarcastic and teasing statements are often taken literally because these children do not get the nonverbal messages of humor conveyed by context and tone due to their difficulties in perceiving emotional prosody.

In conclusion, although children with NVLD have been extensively studied, different results concerning the existence of difficulties in the processing of social information show that further research in this area is needed. Questions exist regarding how much social deficit symptoms are a feature of this disorder; however, as with the other domains (i.e., neuropsychological and academic), their difficulties are more evident when visuospatial processing is involved.

We offer a summary of difficulties and strengths here:

- Difficulties in identifying emotions from body gestures and from adult, but not child, facial expressions
- Weakness in the encoding or interpretation of visual, but not verbal, emotional information

- Similar ability to that of typically developing peers to recognize emotions in some actors, but difficulties in identifying the nonverbal cues (i.e., facial expression, body language, and prosody)
- Difficulties in understanding humor because of the difficulty in interpreting multiple meanings and in perceiving emotional prosody

It should be noted, however, that children with NVLD are mainly characterized by:

- Similar ability as that of typically developing peers to recognize emotions in some actors, but they fail to interpret nonverbal cues
- Children with NVLD are sensitive and mostly generous and altruistic

2.4 Neurological and Anatomical Evidence

At the beginning of this chapter, we cited the "white matter hypothesis" (Rourke, 1995), which highlighted the integrative nature of right hemisphere tasks in comparison to left hemispheric language-based tasks. Rourke theorized that differences in white matter development in NVLD may be the result of prenatal neuronal migration problems. He predicted that children with this disorder, due to their neurological profile, would not make age-appropriate gains in problem solving, concept-formation abilities, and hypothesis testing. On this basis, Rourke hypothesized a relative failure of children with NVLD in making age-appropriate gains in visuoperceptual and problem-solving, mechanical, arithmetic, psychomotor, and tactile-perceptual skills.

Evidence linking the right hemisphere to specific deficits in neurodevelopmental syndromes has been reported by other authors. In the early 1980s, Weintraub and Mesulam (1983) first described patients with a developmental syndrome associated with right hemisphere functioning. These children were characterized as having average intelligence and specific weaknesses in learning (especially in arithmetic), emotional and interpersonal difficulties, visuospatial disturbances, and inadequate paralinguistic communicative abilities. Similarly, Tranel, Hall, Olson, and Tranel (1987) described a group of patients presenting neuropsychological evidence of right hemisphere dysfunction, including severe deficits in nonverbal intelligence, visual memory, and visuospatial functions in the presence of high verbal skills. They concluded that this constellation of symptoms represented a developmental learning disability of the right hemisphere. Evidence concerning this profile in children with NVLD and their social weaknesses was then reviewed by Semrud-Clikeman and Hynd (1990). In a further study, Nichelli and Venneri (1995) reported a 22-year-old man with a developmental profile associated with arithmetic difficulties, visuospatial deficits, and emotional difficulties with intact language abilities. Through neuroimaging techniques, they found a right hemisphere dysfunction in this young man, supporting the claim that this type of learning disability is associated with functional abnormalities of the right hemisphere.

More recently, neuroimaging studies have been conducted to provide evidence in favor of a distinction between NVLD and other neurodevelopmental disorders. Semrud-Clikeman and Fine (2011), studying 28 children with NVLD, found that 25 percent of those children presented unsuspected brain abnormalities, generally including cysts or lesions in the occipital region, while this happened only in 4 percent of children with ASD or typical controls. Other studies found neuroanatomical evidence differentiating NVLD from autism or ADHD. A significantly smaller splenium was found in children with NVLD than in those who had ASD or ADHD, or in typical controls (Fine, Musielak, & Semrud-Clikeman, 2014). Within the NVLD group, those with a smaller splenium fared worse on spatial intelligence measures, whereas this association was not found in the group with autism. In addition, significantly larger volumes of the amygdalae and hippocampi bilaterally were found in a group of children with ASD compared with controls or children with NLD. Moreover, both the children with autism and those with NVLD had smaller left and right anterior cingulate cortex volumes than controls (Semrud-Clikeman et al., 2013). This was the first evidence of children with NVLD differing in some respects from children with autism but possibly sharing the same abnormal connectivity. Finally, Margolis et al. (2019) found that the social deficits common across children with NVLD and autism may derive from distinct alterations in functional connectivity within the salience network supporting social processing. In addition, they have used resting state functional magnetic resonance imaging (fMRI) to show that children with NVLD have reduced global efficiency in the brain's spatial circuit and that such efficiency is associated with social function (Banker et al., 2020a). Lastly, this group has also shown that compared with typically developing children, children with NVLD have reduced left hippocampal volume and greater hippocampal-cerebellar connectivity. Reduced hippocampal volume was associated with worse mathematical problem solving in children with NVLD, and hippocampal functional connectivity was associated with their social function (Banker et al., 2020b).

The studies presented here show that the neuroanatomical evidence for NVLD is emerging. Although at this moment there are only a few studies, the extant research seems to support a visuospatial hypothesis and also seems to show a distinction for NVLD with respect to autism. Hence, from a neurodevelopmental perspective, based on these few studies, NVLD brains do not strongly resemble those with autism. However, in the future, not only neuroimaging studies but also other methods should be used, considering the relationship among behaviors, genetics, and environmental factors that could be involved in shaping the neuropsychological characteristics associated with NVLD. A greater knowledge of the structural aspects of the brains of children with NVLD may help clinicians to understand the causes of specific behavioral difficulties and to differentiate the profiles of children with this disorder from other neurodevelopmental disorders (e.g., ASD or ADHD) to facilitate the differential diagnosis. The correct identification of the disorder would facilitate the choice of a tailored intervention, providing the best aids for these children's needs. In addition, knowledge that a structural difference may be responsible for specific problems may assist parents and teachers in understanding that the child is not willfully misbehaving, reducing negative feelings about them.

Here, we summarize the take away points:

- We are starting to understand how NVLD develops in the brain.
- We may be able to use brain imaging to different DVSD from other similar-seeming disorders.
- We need to educate the public that children are not willfully misbehaving, reducing the misattribution of their motives.

2.5 Conclusions

In this chapter, we have attempted to present an overview of the current research into an understanding of NVLD. This chapter may be more difficult to read than the others, because we used many technical terms. Our goal was to generate further understanding of the challenges of children with DVSD in order to improve their recognition by practitioners, parents, and educators as well as to improve the interventions that they need.

Let us now summarize the most salient points relevant for parents and educators.

Children with NVLD show visuospatial processing deficits that may become evident in academic challenges, mainly mathematics, geometry, handwriting, and science. However, they could encounter difficulties in reading comprehension when inferences about emotional or visuospatial information are required. At school, these children may count on their good verbal abilities to deal with most of these difficulties, and in the following chapters, we will offer more specific suggestions. Regarding social relations with peers, the possibility of having more or less positive experiences will depend on the balance between their difficulties in understanding nonverbal communication and interpreting feelings, and their ability to compensate by using their strength points.

Research findings about the neuropsychological, social, and neuroanatomical aspects may be useful for understanding their general functioning in more and more depth, and all this information may be translated into practical and pragmatic suggestions, as we have tried to do in the next chapters.

Chapter 3

How Is a Developmental Visuospatial Disorder (DVSD) Similar to or Different from Other Disorders?

As seen in the previous chapters, children with a developmental visuospatial disorder (DVSD) may present challenges and/or difficulties in processing visuospatial stimuli, along with a constellation of other symptoms that often make it difficult to differentiate and diagnose which neurodevelopmental disorder (Semrud-Clikeman, Fine, & Bledsoe, 2014) they have. In particular, the DVSD profile overlaps with the clinical profiles of autism spectrum disorders (ASDs), attention-deficit hyperactivity disorder (ADHD), specific learning disorders (with specific impairments in mathematics), developmental coordination disorder, social anxiety, and pragmatic communication disorder. Given the greater popularity of these profiles, the diagnosis of children with DVSD may be confused with them (Cornoldi, Mammarella, & Fine, 2016). However, none of them quite captures the overall pattern of the children's profile, posing problems for the provision of the subsequent intervention strategies and school aids.

In this chapter, we will describe and compare the clinical profiles of children with DVSD and the other clinical profiles reported. Before starting to present similarities and differences between DVSD and other disorders, a reminder of the principal diagnostic characteristics of this disorder appears to be useful in order to have a clear picture of its clinical profile. Children with DVSD often show weaknesses in processing visuospatial information (e.g., difficulties in perceiving organized forms, reproducing drawings, and remembering and manipulating visuospatial information). They also may show fine-motor impairments (e.g., difficulties in drawing, using zippers, and fastening buttons), poor academic achievement (e.g., difficulties in writing, written calculations, geometry, and interpreting graphs), and difficulties in social interaction (e.g., long winded when speaking and interpreting facial expressions) (Cornoldi, Mammarella, & Fine, 2016).

In this chapter, similarities and differences across different clinical profiles will be highlighted in order to better clarify the specific characteristics of each disorder. However, first, let's answer the question of why it is important to distinguish DVSD from other disorders.

Imagine that your child with minor communicative and relational problems, associated with the typical symptoms of DVSD, is instead diagnosed with ASD. It is possible that as parents, you will be confused and will not fully understand why experts have made this diagnosis. At the same time, teachers and clinicians will start to implement standard treatment for autism. Similarly, now imagine your child with DVSD being diagnosed with a specific learning disorder, with impairments in mathematics. Your child will receive specific intervention for improving his/her math skills, but ignoring the other challenges s/he faces in visuospatial abilities and in emotional or social tasks. A more thorough description of the specific characteristics of the DVSD profile would better address the needs and developmental trajectory, and inform the selection of a tailored intervention program for your child. Hence, a correct diagnosis is important, as incorrect diagnoses often result in confusion among the families, the teachers, and the children themselves. In particular, these examples suggest that it is particularly dangerous to emphasize isolated features associated with DVSD (e.g., difficulties social relationships or with mathematics) and ignore other associated problems. For these reasons, in the next sections, we will try to highlight similarities with and differences from other disorders in order to help parents and teachers to be more aware of the main features of children with DVSD.

3.1 Developmental Visuospatial Disorder and Autism Spectrum Disorder

ASDs are characterized by deficits in social communication and social interaction, and obsessive/stereotyped patterns of behavior, interests, or activities (American Psychiatric Association, 2013). The description of the main characteristics of DVSD reported in the previous chapters revealed how this disorder is characterized by overlaps with ASD in behavioral presentations, creating a challenge for its diagnosis (Williams, Goldstein, Kojkowski, & Minshew, 2008).

In particular, the autism profile often confused with DVSD is Asperger syndrome (DSM-IV TR, American Psychiatric Association, APA, 2000) or high functioning autism (DSM-5, APA, 2013). Individuals with this profile demonstrate the impaired social reciprocity and atypical interests and activities seen in autism but show no delays in their early language development (Khouzam, El-Gabalawi, Pirwani, & Priest, 2004).

The similarity between the two disorders is particularly expressed through impairments in motor coordination, in interpersonal awkwardness (Cornoldi et al., 2016; Frith, 1989; Rourke, 1989; Nydén et al., 2010; Volkmar & Klin, 2000), and in pragmatic language difficulties (Landa Klin, Volkmar, & Sparrow, 2000; Rourke & Tsatsanis, 2000). In particular, pragmatic difficulties are characterized by deficits in comprehension of nonverbal social cues (e.g., facial expression, gaze, gesture, and body language), unusual prosody, verbose speech, and difficulties in interpreting jokes and figurative language in conversation (Cornoldi et al., 2016; Ryburn, Anderson, & Wales, 2009; Semrud-Clikeman & Glass, 2008). The autism profile is best diagnosed from a detailed history, school reports, and observing the child. As parents vary in how they report symptoms, one good marker is whether or not the child had engaged in symbolic play as a toddler. Children with autism tend not to play with toys as the "thing" they represent. For example, they may collect fire trucks but not play "fire." Parents may also report that their children use language instrumentally rather than using it to trade ideas. The children do not seem to consider that the "other" may have different ideas.

Discerning the Asperger profile from DVSD is not always easy (Williams et al., 2008). However, it is important to point out that the social impairments reported here are frequently more severe in autism than in DVSD, and in this latter disorder, the restrictive patterns of interest, typical of ASD, are primarily absent (Semrud-Clikeman et al., 2010). Children with DVSD often lack basic social skills; they may stand too close, stare inappropriately or not make eye contact, have a marked lack of concern over appearance, be oblivious to other's reactions, or change topics idiosyncratically. Often, children with DVSD are seen as "odd" children who "just don't get it" socially. They may do better with adults, where they act in a dependent and immature way but may not be seen as "odd." One older view was that Asperger's (now part of ASD) and NVLD were a single disorder that had been given different names by the psychiatric and neuropsychological disciplines, respectively (Korkman, Kemp, & Kirk, 2001; Klin, Volkmar, Sparrow, Cicchetti, & Rourke, 1995). However, Margolis et al. (2019) recently showed that although parents' reported levels of social difficulties did not differ between children with ASD and DVSD, the brain dysfunction underlying such difficulties did differ between the groups. These results point to different neurobiology underlying two distinct disorders.

In Box 3.1, we have tried to summarize the similarities and differences of children with DVSD and autism profiles. As you can see, there are a few similarities, but the disorders also show differences in some features. In particular, concerning social interactions, it is worth noting that usually children with DVSD feel unappreciated by their peers, and although they would like to have social relationships, they do not have the skills to begin and maintain interaction with peers. Moreover, unlike children with the autism profile, their reasoning is more flexible, and they are more open to changing their thoughts and opinions.

Considering visuospatial skills, children with autism may present heterogeneous profiles, showing higher, lower, or comparable

Box 3.1 Similarities and Differences between Children with Developmental Visuospatial Disorder and Autism Spectrum Disorder

Developmental visuospatial disorder vs Autism spectrum disorder

Similarities	*Differences*
Deficits in social interactions	Autism profile: restrictive patterns of interest and obsessive patterns of behavior
Difficulty with the pragmatics of language	Autism profile: literal and inflexible reasoning
	Autism profile: lack of spontaneous sharing of enjoyment and interests with other people
	DVSD profile: visuospatial processing impairments

performance compared with that of children with typical development. A minority of children with the autism profile may show higher verbal and lower visuospatial abilities, but unlike children with DVSD, who, by definition, present a marked deficit in visuospatial intelligence and visuo-constructive abilities, this feature is not consistent in autism. Hence, children with DVSD are expected to perform more poorly in visuospatial tasks (Semrud-Clickeman et al., 2010; Mammarella et al., 2019).

3.2 Developmental Visuospatial Disorder and Attention-Deficit Hyperactivity Disorder

ADHD is a neurobiological developmental disorder characterized by a persistent pattern of inattention and/or hyperactivity/impulsivity interfering with the child's normal psychological development (DSM-5; American Psychiatric Association, 2013). The main problem of children with ADHD is related to their inattention, meaning that they cannot focus their attention for long periods of time and are distracted by irrelevant stimuli in the environment. Impulsivity refers to their tendency to act displaying behaviors characterized by little reflection, while hyperactivity is a state of being unusually active. This disorder is often related to social and relational difficulties (Staikova, Gomes, Tartter, McCabe, & Halperin, 2013). In particular, children with ADHD are often rejected by peers, and the quality of their relationships is inconsistent with their age (Carpenter Rich, Loo, Yang, Dang, & Smalley, 2009). They are also described as immature and having difficulty in creating and maintaining friendships (Hoza et al., 2005).

The presence of attentional problems is also reported in children with DVSD, with particular reference to inattention symptoms (Semrud-Clikeman, 2007). A recent study showed that the most common diagnosis received by children who met criteria for NVLD is ADHD, with the percentage ranging from 33.3 percent to 69.3 percent, depending on the sample considered (see Margolis et al., 2020). It is worth noting that children with DVSD may fail in tasks in which they have to pay attention to visual stimuli, but they often perform well on tasks in which verbal stimuli are presented. On the contrary, children with ADHD have difficulties in maintaining attention to both verbal and visual stimuli (Cornoldi et al., 2016). Previous studies suggested that these attentional difficulties in DVSD are secondary to difficulties in visual-spatial development and visual perceptual problems (Rourke, 2000). The inattention is desultory in DVSD as opposed to distractingly impulsive, as in ADHD. It is as if people with DVSD do not know what to attend to, but once focused, they can sustain attention to detail. The distinction between figure and ground is disturbed, resulting in attention errors.

Difficulties in visuospatial abilities can also occur in children with ADHD. Previous studies highlighted visuospatial working memory and visual attention deficits in children with this disorder (Martinussen et al., 2005; Vance et al., 2007; Willcutt, Doyle, Nigg, Faraone, & Pennington, 2005), while other studies showed average scores in measures of visuospatial intelligence or mental rotation abilities (Semrud-Clickeman et al., 2010; Vance et al., 2007). In addition, a discrepancy between verbal and visuospatial abilities has not been documented within the ADHD population, nor have poor fine-motor skills or difficulties in perceiving organized forms and in reproducing simple drawings by copy or memory (Cornoldi et al., 2016; Semrud-Clickeman et al., 2010a). In Box 3.2, a summary of similarities and differences between these two disorders is presented.

Box 3.2 Similarities and Differences between Children with Developmental Visuospatial Disorder and Attention-Deficit Hyperactivity Disorder

Developmental visuospatial disorder vs Attention deficit hyperactivity disorder

Similarities	*Differences*
Attentional difficulties (specifically with visuospatial stimuli in DVSD)	ADHD profile: impulsivity and hyperactivity
Deficits in social interactions	DVSD profile: rarely shows impulsivity and hyperactivity
	DVSD profile: often characterized by slow processing speed

3.3 Developmental Visuospatial Disorder and Specific Learning Disorders

Specific learning disorders interfere with the ability to learn or use academic skills, such as reading, writing, or arithmetic, which provide the foundations for other, more advanced academic learning (DSM-5; APA, 2013). Specific learning disorders mainly involve reading-related (dyslexia) and math-related (dyscalculia) disorders but may also include deficits in reading comprehension, grammar, and clarity or organization of written expression (Somale, Kondekar, Rathi, & Iyer, 2016). The academic indicators of these disorders may include difficulties in understanding or learning, in reading fluency or written expression, or in the perception/calculation of numbers. Children with these disorders are generally characterized by a worse than expected academic performance.

It is worth noting that children with DVSD often show learning difficulties, in particular in the area of mathematics (Mammarella et al., 2013). Those symptoms are likely to emerge more clearly in the later part of primary school when academic challenges increase. Children with DVSD show strength in verbal activities (e.g., reading decoding and recitation of mathematics facts), and difficulties may be seen in handwriting, conceptual mathematics, geometry, and mathematics-based science. The comorbidity between DVSD and specific learning disorders may be high, and sometimes, a diagnosis of specific learning disorder may be attributed to a child with DVSD. As previously mentioned, the comorbidity between dyscalculia and DVSD is the most frequent. However, the main difference with respect to many cases of a specific mathematics disorder is related to the nature of the impairment. Difficulties in mathematics in children with DVSD are likely the consequence of their visuospatial processing deficits (Mammarella, Lucangeli, & Cornoldi, 2010). Those children usually show problems in spatial representation, placement of values along a number line, aligning columns, carrying and borrowing in written calculations, working with decimals, and omission or rotation of numbers. Often, they do not have problems with mental calculations or with retrieving number facts; thus, simple and automatic skills of calculation are preserved. However, given that many mathematical concepts require visuospatial processing skills, they often obtain poor grades in mathematics. To sum up, some, but not all, children with a DVSD may also meet criteria for a specific learning disorder with impairments in mathematics (see Box 3.3 for similarities and differences between the two disorders).

Overall, in DVSD, learning difficulties are often picked up later than in children with language-based difficulties because children with DVSD are strong decoders and spellers. Inferential reading comprehension is weak relative to decoding and spelling skills. Difficulties in making inferences in language comprehension, in understanding spatial descriptions, and in developing spatial representations by a written text, as well as in understanding humor, have been described (Worling et al., 1999; Semrud-Clikeman & Glass, 2008) in children with DVSD. In other words, their problems in reading comprehension seem to be more specific when visuospatial material is described and when they have to catch the meaning of a concept by observing figures, tables, and diagrams. For these reasons, they may encounter problems in learning science, and generally in organizing complex materials, which is required in secondary schools.

Box 3.3 Similarities and Differences between Children with Developmental Visuospatial Disorder and Specific Learning Disorders

Developmental visuospatial disorder vs Specific learning disorders

Similarities	*Differences*
Mathematics difficulties	Learning disorders profile: difficulties in simple and mechanical aspects of reading or mathematics
Reading comprehension difficulties	DVSD profile: mathematics difficulties as a consequence of visuospatial processing deficits
Deficit in study method and organization	DVSD profile: reading comprehension difficulties only for spatial information (such as in scientific texts)
	DVSD profile: learning difficulties are not specific, and not always the same in children with a DVSD profile, as they depend on visuospatial processing deficits

3.4 Developmental Visuospatial Disorder and Developmental Coordination Disorder

Developmental coordination disorder is characterized by deficits in the acquisition and execution of coordinated motor skills and is manifested by clumsiness and slowness or inaccuracy of performance of motor skills, such as catching objects, riding a bike, or participating in sports, which cause interference with activities of daily living. Hence, in those children, the acquisition and execution of coordinated motor skills is substantially below that expected given the individual's chronological age and opportunity for skill learning and use (DSM-5; APA, 2013).

Unlike other disorders, there are no research studies comparing children with DVSD and developmental coordination disorder, and this is an important limitation of research in this field. However, what research data exist (Durand, 2005; Mammarella & Cornoldi, 2014; Semrud-Clikeman, Walkowiak, Wilkinson, & Christopher, 2010) suggest that children with DVSD can have fine-motor problems, which can become manifest in using scissors, in doing up and undoing buttons, and in handwriting. Thus, it seems that motor problems in children with DVSD are limited to fine-motor skills. In describing the milestones of their development, usually, parents do not remember difficulties in learning to walk. More often, however, they remember that children did not like to play with puzzles, Lego, or drawing. However, Wilkinson-Smith and Semrud-Clikeman (2014) did not find differences in motor speed between children with DVSD and ADHD and concluded that motor speed deficits may not be a defining feature of DVSD. Previous models of NVLD (Rourke, 1995) argued that bilateral deficits in motor speed are primary neuropsychological deficits. However, current research (Cardillo, Vio, & Mammarella, 2020; Mammarella, Cardillo, & Zoccante, 2019) suggests that other types of deficits, such as visuospatial problems, may be more useful in diagnosing DVSD. In addition, it is worth noting that visuospatial skills deficits are not common to all children with developmental coordination disorder (Tsai, Wilson, & Wu, 2008; Alloway & Archibald, 2008) and some research suggests that their ability to mentally rotate images is somewhat intact (Wilson, Maruff, et al., 2004). Thus, visuospatial and motor skills are not exactly the same thing: visuospatial tasks may require fine-motor abilities, but the most important factor is the ability to mentally represent visual and spatial features of an object. By contrast, while visuospatial abilities may be important in motor tasks, spatial mental representations are performed by using the body. Following this reasoning, it is possible that children with DVSD fail in some motor tasks because they are not able to spatially represent how to perform a task with their bodies. Differently, children with developmental coordination disorder may fail in motor tasks, but not necessarily in visuospatial tasks, if motor skills are not involved (see Box 3.4 for a summary of similarities and differences).

Box 3.4 Similarities and Differences between Children with Developmental Visuospatial Disorder and Developmental Coordination Disorder

Developmental visuospatial disorder vs Developmental coordination disorder

Similarities	*Differences*
Fine-motor difficulties	Developmental coordination disorder profile: delayed milestones for gross-motor abilities
Difficulties in copying complex images and in handwriting	Developmental coordination disorder profile: visuospatial skills not necessarily impaired when motor abilities are not required
	DVSD profile: difficulties in mentally representing visual and spatial features of images and objects

3.5 Indefinite Borders among Developmental Disorders

As humans, we naturally want to categorize. However, recent evidence suggests that developmental disorders do not have well-defined boundaries. Although it seems easier to talk about categories when referring to different disorders, such as ADHD, specific learning disorders, and so on, studies of both genetic and environmental risk factors, based on twin designs, familial transmission, or molecular analyses, have raised concerns about the categorical structure of these problems. In particular, neurodevelopmental disorders may be seen on a spectrum, with closely related disorders that have shared symptoms, as well as genetic and environmental risk factors (DSM-5; 2013). Children can and do have multiple disorders and receive more than one diagnosis. Recent research (Margolis et al., 2020), analyzing data from different samples, reported that the most common diagnosis received by children who met criteria for DVSD was ADHD (with the percentage ranging from 69.3 percent to 33.3 percent), followed by anxiety disorder (from 32.9 percent to 13.3 percent) and specific learning disorder (13.1 percent). To complicate the matter, children frequently change during development; not only do they grow up, but also, their symptoms may change according to the requirements of their environment. For this reason, some disorders (thanks to scientific evidence) have been described with developmental trajectories. For example, a child with ADHD may (or may not) become an adult with an anxiety disorder, and this depends on several external as well as individual factors during development (Thomas & Ollendick, 2008). In other words, not every child with ADHD will develop an anxiety disorder, but in some conditions, such as without interventions, this could happen.

To sum up, each developmental disorder is characterized by specific features; however, some symptoms may be present also in other disorders. In addition, we must take into account how the specific characteristics of the children, their families, and their environment may create the conditions for different developmental trajectories.

In this chapter, we have tried to define similarities and differences among different but similar disorders. In order to underline and better illustrate the complexity of developmental disorders, we will present the case of Christine (her name and identifying information have been altered to protect her identity). We are describing Christine because she first received a diagnosis of DVSD, not meeting any of the criteria for autism, but when she grew up and met the additional social challenges of a teenager, new symptoms appeared, which could have complicated the diagnostic process. When we met Christine for the first time, she was an eighth-grade girl whose parents were concerned about her math performance. She had above average overall intelligence with higher verbal than visuospatial reasoning skills. On the neuropsychological measures, she clearly had the pattern of visuospatial processing deficits. For example, she was not able to copy complex geometrical figures by drawing and showed poor math performance, while language skills were intact. She did not have any problems with inferential comprehension in reading. At this time, ASD was not even a consideration. She had had good friends through primary school and felt herself to be part of her peer group. Symbolic play development had been normal, and she exhibited no repetitive behaviors. Thus, it was determined that she met the diagnostic criteria for a diagnosis of DVSD.

Her parents returned when Christine was 14 years old. She was now isolated from her peers, who complained that she was too literal. Often, she had difficulties in writing papers; in particular, she tended to write lists and utilized less integrated sentences than her peers. She maintained the specific features of the DVSD, but now, there were more difficult and advanced peer and academic demands that highlighted her weaknesses in social perception and inferential reasoning. Given her previous history of good social adjustment, one would still never diagnose her with ASD. We would understand her social issues as components of her DVSD. However, her socio-relational difficulties at that age easily could resemble a much milder form, or at least, some symptoms looked more similar to those observed in high functioning autism. Had she not already had a thorough neurological examination, her accurate diagnosis might have been missed.

This case of a complex relationship between DVSD and some symptoms more typical of the autism profile may be an example of how categorizing too rigidly can confuse, rather than clarify, our thinking. As previously mentioned, according to the demands of the environment, several latent problems may become more evident; by contrast, some strengths could also emerge with development. For all these reasons, it is crucial to have a complete neurological exam and monitor continuously how symptoms change when children grow up, and how they are able to adapt and to cope with the demands of the environment.

Chapter 4

Managing Developmental Visuospatial Disorder (or Nonverbal Learning Disability) at School

Tips for Teachers

Children with developmental visuospatial disorder (DVSD) may face hurdles or impediments in a variety of different life contexts, such as in the school community, where the challenges faced will shift and increase as the work load and productivity demands increase. Therefore, our children with DVSD need to be supported in school with specific and appropriate interventions and educational strategies based on their developmental level and taking account of the environmental context. Unfortunately, we currently have only a modest amount of scientific evidence on the efficacy of interventions for children with nonverbal learning disability. In other words, the scientific literature on interventions is scarce in this field.

However, in this chapter, we will offer an overview of optimal learning environments and of how one might develop or adapt interventions that have been previously mentioned in the literature by specifically considering the school settings. In addition, we will provide some suggestions for teachers and parents on how to help children with DVSD best succeed at school.

Toward that end, we stress the importance of finding a school environment that will maximize our students' overall success. We hope that school administrations can become more open-minded, flexible, and willing to consider the specific unique needs of the whole child, not just their disability and remediation needs; recognizing, supporting, and enhancing their strengths as well as their challenges. It is important to find a school environment that reduces the chances of shame and confusion for the child with DVSD. Collaboration is also key, as a school that is comfortable with a team approach is required, given the many types of interventions students with DVSD will often utilize (Broitman et al., 2020). Considering the difficulties of these students with spatial orientation and some motor skills, when possible, the school should attempt to reduce the number of transitions for the student, such as fewer trips to the locker, fewer classroom changes, etc., as well as help to open their lockers and change quickly for gym. Books and supplies should be arranged such that there will be no need to go back and forth to get items. They should also provide a simplified map of the school and guidance on getting to specialists and arranging a buddy system.

Students with DVSD often exhibit inattention. For this reason, preferential seating should be allowed, and when possible, students should sit near and facing the teacher/front row, not close to behaviorally challenged children or children who are noisy or fidgety. Because the learning styles of students with DVSD are concrete and literal, they will be helped by having very specific directions and using rubrics (scoring criteria). These can be very effective, as they plot the direction that needs to be taken, specifically guiding the learner to broader skill development in a very concrete, specific fashion. It's also helpful to front-load expectations, remind children of context, and review their prior knowledge. Multi-tasking can provide additional stress and should not be required. Additional time is useful during any transitions, and ample warning prior to requiring a shift in attention is helpful.

Teachers should be willing to have less visual distraction on walls/boards. Students with DVSD benefit more from the use of verbal rather than visual contents. Thus, it is useful to privilege verbal explanations in the transmission of content and also in the presentation/resolution of problems, as well as for different indications.

Handwriting could be challenging for these students. For this reason, they should not be required to listen and write at the same time. Classroom notes should be emailed home in advance when possible, especially providing notes ahead of lectures in the upper grades. Provide handouts, notes, and outlines for the student instead of requiring copying from the board. When the blackboard is used, employ a consistent visual spatial format for organizing information on the blackboard. Pre-teaching and reviewing instructional content are also suggested, with the warning to be cautious and make sure that generalization has taken place. Formal cooperative learning can be successful, but only if care is taken in arranging the makeup of the groups (Molenaar-Klumper, 2002).

Because of difficulty in visual tracking, teachers should be open to reducing information on a page and use a flip chart to separate concepts when needed. When assessing the student, teachers should agree to stress content and accuracy in presentations rather than spending too much time on visual appearance (Broitman et al., 2020). They should allow the student many opportunities to present information verbally through oral presentations as long as the student is comfortable with this. Because the student may tend to lose their place during a test, it is useful if the school/teacher allows the student to write answers directly on the test sheet rather than requiring them to use a separate answer sheet. Teachers should be aware of the difficulty associated with visual tasks such as matching. Teachers should simplify test answer sheet layouts and the arrangement of visual–spatial math assignments (no credit should be lost for a correct answer placed in the wrong column or space). Whenever possible, the use of graph paper is recommended to keep columns aligned in written math assignments. Teachers should allow the use of a calculator for math-related activities.

Both public and private schools can be options for the child with DVSD, depending on the level of cooperation and what accommodations or modifications are allowed. In some states, individualized educational programs (IEPs) may be provided at school, which are individualized plan that establish the educational goals for eligible students with difficulties in different learning domains for one school year. However, because DVSD is not yet a recognized diagnosis, the child's classification for special education services will have to be based on some other diagnosis (Broitman et al., 2020).

4.1 General Intervention Guidelines for Children with DVSD

"Treat early and often" is the commonly heard refrain, as most professionals believe that children with DVSD can and will learn, but it will take repeated, continual, and specific interventions (Tsatsanis & Rourke, 2003). Evidence suggests that the earlier and more accurate the diagnosis, coupled with early intervention, the better the outcome (Martin, 2007; Thompson, 1997).

The general guidelines that we will present here may be partly applied also to other neurodevelopmental disorders, but to be more specific to the case of DVSD, they have been inspired by previous guidelines (see Broitman et al., 2020; Broitman & Davis, 2013; Cornoldi, 1997; Cornoldi, Mammarella, & Fine, 2016; Davis & Broitman, 2011; Tsatsanis & Rourke, 2003), literature (Foss, 1991; Matte & Bolaski, 1998), and our own experience. These guidelines contain general principles and suggestions that can be utilized with the aid of an expert practitioner.

Children with DVSD benefit from direct, systematic, and structured instructions, similarly to other students with learning disabilities. Within this general framework, there are specific principles that may be useful for these children (see Box 4.1). In particular,

Box 4.1 Guidelines for Intervention on Children with DVSD (Mainly Derived by Cornoldi, Mammarella & Fine, 2016)

General Intervention Guidelines for Children with DVSD

1. Define a long-term intervention plan for supporting the child with DVSD and identify a clinician who will assume the responsibility for its coordination.
2. Establish priorities, working on one or two things at a time; do not "overload."
3. Use a multimodal approach intervening on the child and on the school, family, and social contexts.
4. Develop awareness in the child of their specific strengths and weaknesses, helping them to build the capacity for self-understanding and self-advocacy.
5. Accept the idea that it will be impossible to eliminate some specific deficits and look for ways in which those modalities that negatively affect the child's general development can be minimized or avoided.
6. Work to prevent the development of secondary symptoms, in particular related to emotional and socio-relational difficulties, minimizing shame.
7. Within a developmental perspective, optimize cognitive skills early on and build on adaptive skills in older children.
8. Help the child to interpret nonverbal communication signs.
9. Increase appropriate self-efficacy and self-effort attributions in order to motivate the child to efforts for change and reduce the risks for learned helplessness.
10. Suggest alternative strategies, and help the child to think of alternative strategies for coping.
11. Develop verbal strategies for specific situations where the child is in difficulty.
12. Automatize basic procedural knowledge in the areas of difficulty.
13. Avoid a memory overload, specifically on visuospatial materials.
14. Divide complex tasks into sub-objectives and aid the child to use verbal self-instructions.

due to the risk of impairments in adaptive functioning, a long-term intervention plan is recommended. It should be supervised by a clinician who can systematically interact with the different practitioners who will interact with the child throughout the course of their development. Generally speaking, during the life of the child, specific interventions should be tailored to the present challenges of the child, but also considering and anticipating the most serious problems the child is likely to face during each different stage of development. Thus, it seems important to establish priorities for the intervention and support children with regard to wellness, self-efficacy, and awareness of their own problems. The financial burdens for families must also be considered and utilized to assist in prioritization and allocation of funds.

Overall, children with DVSD, as with other specific neuropsychological problems, benefit from interventions based on the logic of the deficit-centered training (i.e., training activities focused on their main difficulty based on their profile). Our clinical experience suggests that during primary school, it is best to focus interventions on visuospatial and visuo-motor skills. In addition, during this developmental period, given the importance and impact that academic success has on children's development and adaptation, interventions should focus on mastering specific skills in the academic areas (mathematics, reading comprehension, and written expression). In addition, in order to promote psychological adjustment and/or social interaction skills, assertiveness training, interpersonal problem solving, creative drama, and cognitive-behavioral therapy may be useful during the pre-adolescence period.

In order to maximize the efficacy of an intervention for a child with DVSD, one should consider all the potential areas or possibilities for improving the child's quality of life. Interventions might include medication to reduce symptoms of anxiety, depression, or inattention. A good plan must necessarily be directed not only to the child but also to school and family. In order to choose the best intervention at a particular time for a specific child with this profile, we suggest a consultation with an expert psychologist or practitioner who can refer to the child's specific neurological profile. Beside specific interventions, some suggestions for an integrated intervention should be provided to teachers and families, and we will present such recommendations in the next paragraphs.

4.2 Academic Area of Intervention in Children with DVSD

The school setting is particularly important, because frequently it is in this environment that the main problems of children with DVSD emerge, therefore providing a crucial opportunity for effective intervention. Moreover, as children spend most of their time at school, it is essential to address their psychological problems and academic skill deficits. Improving competence in academically impaired areas may require some activities that occur at school (either individually or in the context of the classroom) and others that must be necessarily carried out after school within an extra-curricular environment. In this regard, in Italy, there is a long tradition of interventions for children with DVSD, and for example, in 1997 Cornoldi et al. published a large volume including practical activities developed for improving difficulties in several areas (reported here) in which the challenges of children with DVSD are taken into account:

- Visuospatial memory and visuospatial abilities
- Drawing
- Handwriting
- Arithmetic
- Geography
- Science
- Social skills

Overall, academic interventions are often needed to support children in several subjects, such as mathematics, writing, and planning/organization. In addition, as previously mentioned, social and emotional interventions may be useful to improve functioning at home and school and to support resiliency into adulthood. As for academic interventions in children with DVSD, we repeat that there is no available research to support the efficacy of these interventions. Thus, the strategies suggested here are derived from clinical reports and experience by considering the profile of strengths and deficits seen in children with DVSD.

We offer in the following some general suggestions, which could be useful to teachers in the school setting, and then follow with specific suggestions for the most critical areas of academic intervention.

First of all, it is important that teachers become aware of the main problems that children with DVSD may encounter at school, but also note that their good verbal abilities offer an important strength to balance their difficulties. Some modifications of the classroom may be useful: for example, given their difficulties in spatial orientation, modified schedules and signage (e.g., exit, gym ...) could be used at school, such as using modified wooden clocks that clearly point out the initial and final periods of an activity. Children with DVSD could benefit from pre-learning using the teachers' notes, which would help them anticipate the general ideas and follow the basic outline in a lecture. Moreover, diagrams, tables, graphs, and complex figures should be used minimally; when they are necessary, the teacher should verbally explain their meaning very carefully. For testing their achievement, oral exams should be preferred to written tests, as students with DVSD are more often characterized by good verbal abilities, and they are usually able to verbally explain what they have learned. When scoring their written exams, they should not be penalized because of poor handwriting skills, and laptops should be utilized as much as possible to increase the readability of their work. Extra time should also be provided for tests, as their handwriting is frequently slow. Thus, activities with scissors, set squares, and rulers, and more generally drawing and handwriting, should be limited or facilitated for students with this profile. In addition, they need help in organizing their schoolbag, in taking notes, in recalling homework and commitments, and in checking to see that follow up has occurred. Many a child's perfectly done assignment has remained on the kitchen table! Moreover, in physical education and sports activities during school time, teachers should pay particular attention to decide whether the activity is appropriate for the child with DVSD or whether they need a modification or adaptation to the school curriculum.

Overall, teacher-modeled problem solving is important for teaching students with DVSD. This method—also called cognitive apprenticeship—is based on the observation of an expert working on a task (Collins, Brown, & Newman, 1988) through verbal mediation or "think out loud." In particular, teaching methods that integrate spatial and verbal processes are useful in helping students to integrate their verbal strengths with their areas of weakness. For example, in drawing a figure, the child may improve his performance by verbally describing the figure prior to and during drawing it. Similarly, in order to improve the ability to put numbers in columns to perform written calculations, children may be helped first by consulting simple written instructions and then by using verbal self-instructions (see Van Luit & Van de Rijt, 2009). As previously mentioned, children with DVSD often encounter difficulties in interpreting tables, figures, and graphs. For this reason, tables and graphs should be described verbally in order to help children to integrate the presented information. In addition, children with DVSD may not be helped by conceptual maps or diagrams for studying written materials. Teachers should suggest summaries and key-words instead of conceptual maps (Mammarella & Lipparini, 2015). In summary, teaching explicit and systematic cognitive strategies may be useful for children with DVSD (see Box 4.2). Teachers may suggest that the child writes down strategies that were previously successful so that he or she can refer to these strategies when needed.

Many students with DVSD are found to have difficulty with receptive language, or the ability to understand words and language challenges, especially in the areas of pragmatic language or the social language skills that we use in our daily interactions with others. Others have written about how these difficulties can impact aspects of advanced reading skills that depend on such abilities, such as inferencing, summarizing, and saliency determination (Worling, Humphries, & Tannock, 1999; Cardillo, Basso Garcia, Mammarella, & Cornoldi, 2018). And again, these challenges can be remediated with direct and explicit reading comprehension instruction.

Finally, children with DVSD are often less competent than peers in social skills; hence, during playtime, particular attention should be placed to avoiding the risk of isolation, teasing, and bullying. For example, teachers could offer ways to manage these situations and suggestions on who to ask for help if necessary. In Box 4.2, we have summarized the main areas of intervention at school for children with DVSD.

Depending on the school grade attended by children, teachers can implement different educational adaptations. Box 4.3 summarizes possible educational adaptations for students with DVSD depending on their grade level.

In the following sections, we will consider separately the most crucial areas of intervention (mathematics, writing, and social abilities) for children with DVSD.

We begin with the two primary academic areas typically requiring attention for children with DVSD, which are mathematics and writing. Interventions in these areas can consist of direct instruction and specific interventions, modification of the classroom

Box 4.2 Environmental Modifications and Possible Curriculum Adaptation for Students with DVSD

Grade level	*Environmental modifications*	*Curriculum modifications*
Kindergarten (<6 y)	Clear use of signage (e.g., exit, toilet...) and written and verbalized schedules and itineraries reduce stimulation and lighting issues	Pre-teach basic outlines offer oral explanations
Primary school (6–12 y)	Use adapted wall clocks in classroom Supervise break and playtime in order to reduce risk of isolation and bullying	Limit or simplify activities with scissors, set squares, and other instruments Use concrete examples and use manipulatives to illustrate concepts
Secondary school (12–16 y)	Minimize transitions between classes Duplicate materials, leaving a second set at home Assignments listed on the web Offer ways to manage social or complex situations with individual or group treatment	Verbally explain the meaning of graphs, diagrams, and complex figures Teaching explicit and systematic strategies to "think out loud" Take care of the student during the assignments, and in taking note of homework activities, using scaffolding strategies and/or overseeing them Utilize oral exams instead of written evaluation

Box 4.3 Educational Adaptations for Students with DVSD

Grade level	*Educational*
Kindergarten (<6 y)	- adaptation of visuo-constructive activities (e.g., simplified puzzles and drawings ...)
Primary school (6–12 y)	- adaptation of physical education and sports (i.e., by modifying instructions and providing support equipment) - adaptation in playing instruments - adaptation in drawing (i.e., provision of hand grips for paintbrushes and pencils) - adaptation in mathematics (i.e., providing sheets with guided spaces to line up columns in written calculations)
Secondary school (12–16 y)	- adaptation in mathematics (i.e., create special pages for students with a few problems visible at a time) - adaptation in drawing (i.e., simplification/ reduction of tasks involving visual–spatial skills) - adaptation in physics and chemistry (i.e. providing the student guided notes to fill in during the lesson) - adaptation in reading comprehension and handwriting (i.e., For complex reading tasks, it can be useful to write notes in the margin to help the student focus on certain points. Providing adapted worksheets to reduce the need for handwriting, asking for "Circle the answer" or "Fill in the white space")

environment, modification of academic load, and scaffolding to support the student's progress in non-affected areas.

4.3 Mathematics

In the area of mathematics, children with DVSD may perform differentially on different types of tasks. Forrest (2004; see also Mammarella, Lucangeli, & Cornoldi, 2010) found that children with this profile may draw on their considerable verbal ability to perform language-based math skills adequately, such as retrieving simple calculations from their long-term memory. Written mathematics was found to be most impaired, suggesting that the mechanics of performing written math (i.e., lining up number columns, carrying and borrowing procedures) is an area of difficulty. Modifications to help with this problem include using graph or column paper to assist with number alignment (see Figure 4.1). Adjustment of the curriculum to include an enriched verbal explanation of the material as opposed to blackboard demonstration only has proved useful according to clinical report (Davis, J.M. personal communication). While early number concepts and facts may not necessarily pose difficulty, children with DVSD may benefit from one-on-one tutoring by a mathematics educator skilled in translating math concepts verbally as concepts become more abstract and spatial (geometry, trigonometry). The use of a calculator for math-related activities should be allowed.

Overall, given that one of the strength areas of children with DVSD is represented by verbal abilities, teachers should encourage these children to use verbal strategies when visuospatial material is presented. For example, there are curricula available in North America that take a verbal or narrative approach to mathematics. For example, *Life of Fred Mathematics* (Stanley Schmidt, Ontario, Canada) uses simple but entertaining stories to teach mathematics from elementary to university levels, covering calculus and statistics. Other approaches to mathematics emphasize mental calculation, teaching concepts without a strong demand for writing. One example of this type of approach is the *Verbal Math Lesson* series that covers basic mathematical concepts, fractions, and percentages (Levin & Langton, Mountcastle Company). Another example is *On Cloud Nine®* (Tuley & Bell, 1997), which stimulates the ability to image and verbalize the concepts underlying math processes.

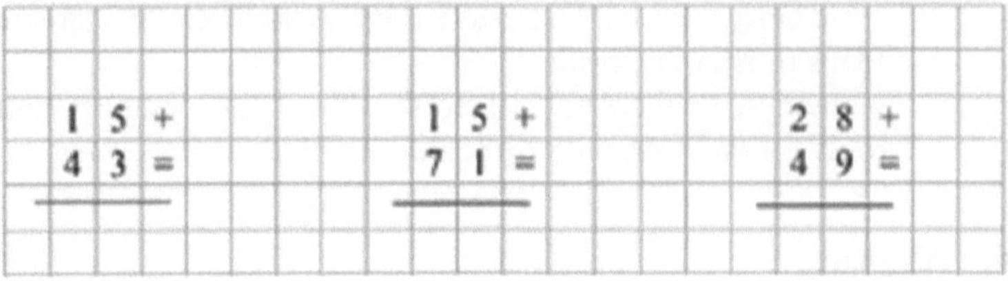

Figure 4.1 Example of adaptation to assist children with column numbers alignment.

Concept and numeral imagery are integrated with language and applied to math computation and problem solving.

Overall, the main suggestions for helping children with DVSD that teachers should consider are summarized as follows:

- Simplify complex abstract activities into several steps in order to help the child to apply procedures and information already learned
- Promote the comprehension of mathematical rules and concepts by using verbal abilities
- Reinforce mental calculation and simple arithmetical facts that the child can easily learn
- Help the student to use explicit verbal self-instruction for guiding the solution of written calculations or word problems
- Use simple visual supports, for example, putting numbers in columns
- Provide printed geometric figures when geometrical word problems are presented
- Prioritize learning of functional skills for solving problems in real life
- Use math apps – see following examples:
    - Mathmagics (https://apps.apple.com/us/app/mathemagics-mental-math/id306586847): App designed for learning and practicing tricks of mental calculation.
    - Desmos (www.desmos.com/calculator/dseyqv1dde) or Geogebra (https://tube.geogebra.org/): Both allow you to drag points, lines, and circles around to see how they behave as the measure of angles and line segments changes.
    - Modmath (www.modmath.com): App displays virtual graph paper, which kids can use to set up math equations. Kids enter their equations; the program aligns numbers and symbols in neat columns and/or rows so the equations are clearly legible. They save their worksheets and create PDFs to share or print.
    - www.dyscalculia.org/math-tools offers a range of apps and tools for children with difficulties in mathematics learning.

4.4 Writing

Writing is an area of difficulty both for beginning writers and as children advance through school. Initially, the physical act of writing can be a barrier to developing handwriting as a method of effective communication. Children with DVSD may need specific interventions to develop fine-motor control (see Figure 4.2). Handwriting Without Tears ® (www.hwtears.com) has been used with some success in schools, according to clinical report.

When the physical act of writing is severely challenging, moving the child to a keyboard-based system is advised. The keyboard should not take the place of learning how to handwrite; however, when writing is required for content rather than practice, it is important to allow the child to demonstrate their knowledge. The use of a computer word processor is highly recommended for written school assignments, because the spatial and fine-motor skills needed for typing are not as complicated as those involved in handwriting. Even dictation is recommended for content-based exercises if the child is not able to produce a written product. By allowing the child to continue to grow academically without being held back by production issues, some negative emotionality and lowering of self-esteem may be avoided.

Older students may experience difficulty with organizing their ideas into a cohesive written report (see Figure 4.3). If symptoms of ADHD are present, this type of task can become even more challenging. Software programs such as Inspiration® and Kidspiration® (Inspiration Software, 2008) help students develop report ideas using webs, which are then converted into outline form. Finally, adolescents with DVSD may need more help from adults during this process than do their non-affected peers.

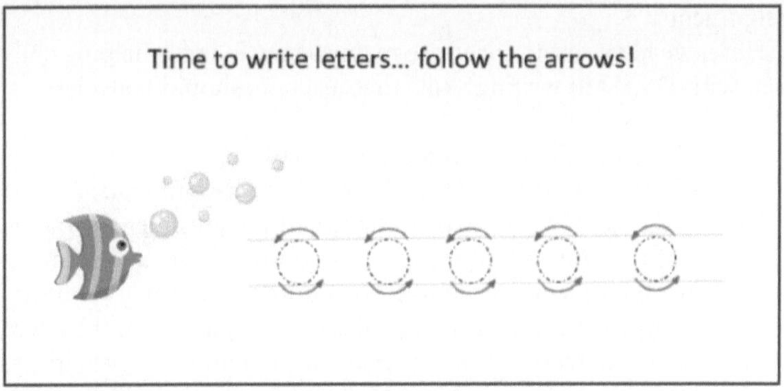

Figure 4.2 Example of an activity supporting fine-motor control and writing.

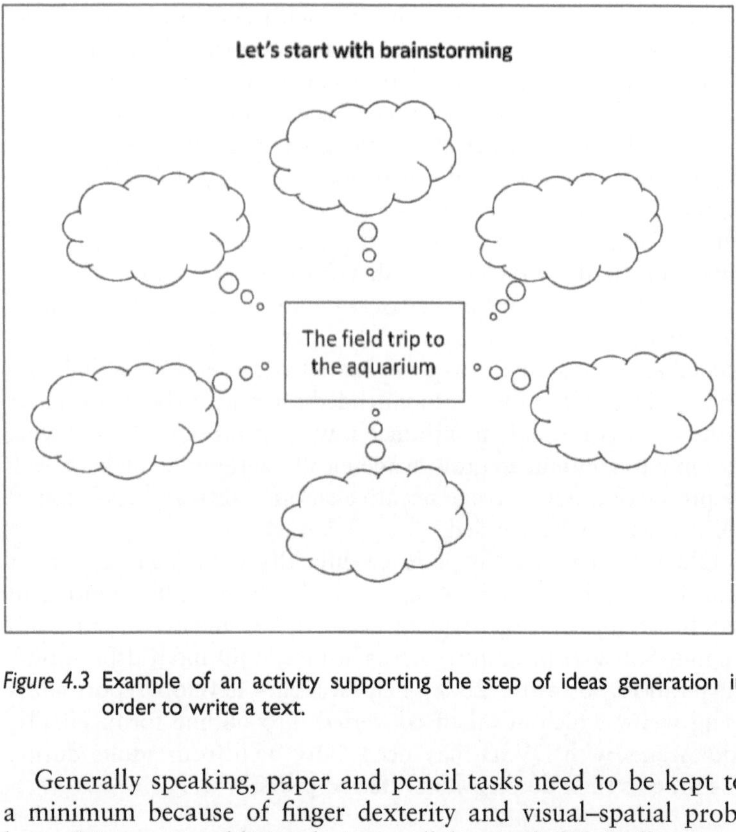

Figure 4.3 Example of an activity supporting the step of ideas generation in order to write a text.

Generally speaking, paper and pencil tasks need to be kept to a minimum because of finger dexterity and visual–spatial problems. Moreover, additional time will be needed for all written assignments.

Here, we have summarized the main suggestions for helping children with DVSD in writing skills that teachers should consider:

- Paper and pencil tasks need to be limited.
- Additional time will be needed for written assignments.
- When the homework involves handwriting, consider the possibility of recommending the use of a computer word processor.
- When the student is required to produce a written composition, suggest they: (a) generate ideas (see Figure 4.3), (b) select the most important ideas, (c) create a plan and organize ideas, (d) write according to the plan, and (e) review the written composition.

- In the following, we have reported some useful apps:
  - The Writing Revolution: Judith C. Hochman and Natalie Wexler (www.thewritingrevolution.org/). Using The Writing Revolution method can be a way of ensuring that DVSD students are grasping content and thinking analytically. Provides a clear method of instruction to use across grades and courses. May improve reading comprehension, improve organizational and study skills, enhance speaking abilities, and help develop analytical capabilities.
  - Story Builder (www.thesmartfeed.com/creations/story-builder): helps children to 1) improve paragraph formation; 2) improve integration of ideas; and 3) improve higher-level abstractions by inference.
  - Simple Mind+ (https://simplemind.eu/): mind mapping for any kind of writing project. Students use the app to brainstorm or organize ideas on a specific topic.

4.5 Social Skills

Another crucial role of the school is to mitigate and help cope with the social interaction problems of children with DVSD. Shyness and social isolation may occur, as well as social rejection or bullying by their peers (Tanguay, 2001). Young children and pre-adolescents may meet difficulties in interacting with classmates and in particular with groups of children of the same age and of the same gender, looking for individual friends or for interactions with groups of different ages. In adolescence, the problem may be also complicated by the child's difficulty in interacting with peers of the opposite gender. However, friendships with others are important for children with DVSD. Teachers can take a leading role in creating supervised situations where the child interacts with other children. Despite the fact that researchers have not specifically considered the case of DVSD, there is robust evidence that supervised peer tutoring and cooperative learning may be effective with children with social or learning difficulties (Jordan & Métais, 1997; Goodwin, 1999). Other useful strategies include giving specific responsibilities within the learning community to the child (Lavoie, 1994). Examples of this might include being a time-keeper and participating in organized groups such as collaborating for the class or school newspaper.

Moreover, direct teaching of social perception skills through practice, modeling, and role-playing may be helpful. Teaching social perception through task analysis and rule teaching allows the child with DVSD to verbally process the information and use his/her strengths to learn new skills. It is worth noting that the intervention needs to progress slowly with plenty of structure and time for the child to practice foundational skills before moving on to the more complex activities that require the building of trust in order to attempt them.

Generally, interventions include those involving parents, the social skills curriculum (including coaching and friendship groups), and a group-based intervention based on learning about emotions and social applications. For generalization of skills to occur, parent and teacher involvement are important in order to allow practice of newly learned skills. One of the weaknesses of these interventions, however, is the lack of empirical validation for children with DVSD.

In the following, the main suggestions for helping children with DVSD that teachers should take into account are summarized.

- Social skills need to be addressed very specifically. They will need to be taught like any other academic subject and infused as part of all other subject areas. Students should have an entire section of their IEP dedicated to social skill goals.
- When groups are being formed in the general education classroom or for other activities (i.e., sports), the groups should be assigned so as to limit the social isolation students may feel by being chosen last for a group.
- It is important to place students in a group with peers who will not be critical of them but who will encourage their active participation in the group.
- Because of the likelihood of the students associating with peers who are in trouble, their caregivers should make sure they are supervised. Other suggestions include getting them involved in an organized activity to increase contact with appropriately social peers.
- Pair students with DVSD with an older student to learn appropriate behaviors and improve social skills and functioning at school.
- To bolster their social skills with same-aged peers, children should participate in a social skills group of same-aged and gendered peers. This may be done with the school counselor and with children from their classroom and other classrooms in their grade level.

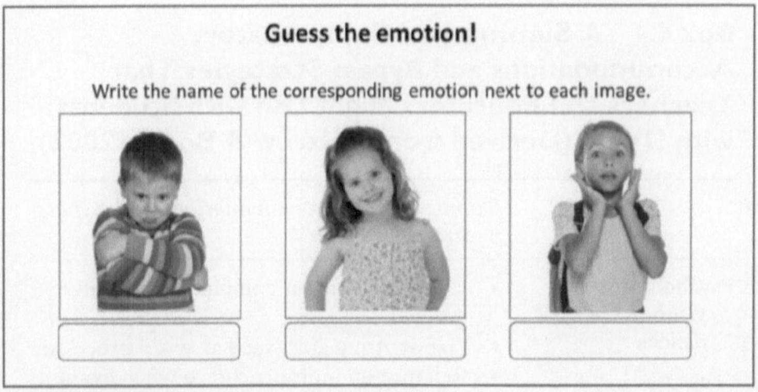

Figure 4.4 Example of an activity used to learn and practice the comprehension of facial emotional expression.

- Facilitate social relationships with peers by using role-play and practice to elicit positive interactions.
- Social awareness should be cultivated, focusing on the relevant aspects of given situations and pointing out the irrelevancies. Discrepancies between the individual's perceptions regarding a situation and the perceptions of others should be made explicit.
- The meaning of eye contact, gaze, and various inflections—as well as tone of voice, facial and hand gestures, non-literal communications such as humor, figurative language, irony, sarcasm, and metaphor—should all be taught, with all elements being made verbally explicit and appropriately and repeatedly drilled (see Figure 4.4).
- Techniques such as practicing in front of a mirror, listening to recorded speech, watching a video-recorded behavior, and so forth should all be incorporated.
- It is important to help the student develop the ability to make inferences, to predict, to explain motivation, and to anticipate multiple outcomes so as to increase the flexibility with which the student both thinks about and uses language.

In Box 4.4 some compensatory instruments that can be used by teachers based on the characteristics of the child with DVSD and the academic areas of difficulty are reported.

Box 4.4 A Summary of Compensatory Accommodations and Bypass Strategies That Teachers and Educators Might Use with Students with DVSD (Derived from Telzrow & Bonar, 2002)

	Compensatory Accommodations and Bypass Strategies
Psychomotor and visuo-perceptual deficits	• Extended time for completion of written tasks • Handwriting aids, such as word processor • Reliance on multiple choice when examining content knowledge • Organizing worksheets with a limited number of clear, well-spaced prompts • Use of oral or written directions and explanations instead of visual maps and schemas
Arithmetic difficulties	• Graph paper to assist in column alignment when completing arithmetic problems • Color-coded arithmetic worksheets to cue left–right directionality • Commercially or teacher-prepared chapter summaries and study guides
Social interaction deficits	• Support students in incorporating their strengths and passions when selecting their career path • Choosing structured, adult-directed, individual, or single-peer social activities over unstructured or large group events

Finally, schools must support making modifications and accommodations in the school curriculum as needed for the child with DVSD. In many countries, vocational guidance is also an assumed responsibility of the school. Guidance that takes care to understand the individual strengths and weaknesses of the child with DVSD will be important in guiding him or her to vocations aligned with their interests as well as their skills.

Chapter 5

Living with Developmental Visuospatial Disorder (or Nonverbal Learning Disability) at Home

The Role of Parents

5.1 Parenting a Child with Developmental Visuospatial Disorder

Parenting a child with developmental visuospatial disorder (DVSD) or nonverbal learning disability can present both rewards and challenges. Children with DVSD can find fulfilling and rewarding life paths, but getting them there can present difficulties. One in particular, which we mentioned in the previous chapters, is that unlike other neurodevelopmental disorders, such as ADHD, or specific learning disorders, there is not a recognized diagnostic category for DVSD. This is because at this moment, the DVSD profile has not been inserted into the international diagnostic systems. We are hopeful that this will be remedied in the future and applaud the efforts of Dr. Prudence Fisher and her colleagues at Columbia University. However, due to the diagnostic confusions, these children have often received many different diagnoses at different ages from practitioners, which creates misunderstanding and uncertainty in families. Parents do not understand what the main problem of their child is, and are often confused about how to help them. The difficulties of the child may be misunderstood at school, and the child frequently experiences rejection from their peers. "It is hard to have difficulty with tasks that are generally considered to be enjoyable. It is isolating to not be able to connect with activities that peers love. Sometimes I needed to pretend to like things that were hard for me. I feared that not liking them meant I was inadequate" wrote Brett Mills in recalling his experience (Broitman & Davis, 2013, p. 328; to learn more about Brett's experience, see Broitman et al. (2020). Brett's thoughts help us to understand the feeling of a child with DVSD and the consequences to their self-esteem due to not being accepted and understood by peers.

In addition, teachers, in most cases, have no idea what DVSD is and how to help children with such problems. The presence of multiple and different diagnoses, as mentioned before, is not a support. In a research published in 2016 (Mammarella et al., 2016), we found that children with DVSD suffered more school anxiety than children with typical development and children with a diagnosis of dyslexia. In our view, this finding may be due in part to the poor knowledge of this profile. Consequently, we hypothesized that children might be handled inappropriately at school; in other words, cases of DVSD may go undetected and teachers may be unable to recognize the disorder promptly. An inappropriate approach to these children may make them feel inadequate and anxious about their performance at school. A generally poor understanding of the symptoms typical of children with DVSD could also be responsible for parents misattributing their child's struggles and behaviors, resulting in a lack of appropriate attunement, which would further contribute to the children's anxiety, particularly as regards their academic achievements. In fact, a study by Antshel and Joseph (2006) on mothers of 8- to 11-year-old children with nonverbal learning disability, with dyslexia, and with typical development found that the mothers of children with nonverbal learning disability reported higher levels of dysfunctional interactions with their children than in the case of the other two groups. However, as Broitman et al. (2020) point out, "Parents can be taught how to deal with their own frustrations, understand their limitations, and realize that their own family histories and dynamics will influence the expectation they have for their children. Parents can be shown the additional complicated impact these expectations will have on children with Nonverbal learning disability. Making the link between parental frustration and the message it gives their child can be very useful."

Hence, given the difficulties families may encounter in having a child with DVSD, what can be suggested?

As emphasized previously in this chapter and elsewhere, parents need a thorough evaluation of their child in order to know which kind of support is necessary. Every child is different, and although there is a typical profile of children with DVSD, points of strength and weakness may change, not only according to the age of the child but also among individuals. When parents have a clear picture of these points, actual acts of accurate advocacy can begin. We offer a variety of suggestions to help families navigate these complexities. Our initial suggestions are listed here.

- *Know the rules, as in the appropriate laws and policies.* Every country has different laws; hence, we cannot take this point into account in detail, but we strongly believe that it is a crucial aspect to consider. School and family support depend on the specific policies of each country, and families of children with neurodevelopmental disorders, in general, and DVSD in particular, should understand what services they are entitled to and that they could require for their child. For example, as explained in Broitman et al. (2020), in America, IEPs are developed, based upon psychoeducational evaluations, in order to develop appropriate interventions. This can be very hard to obtain for students with DVSD, as the diagnosis is not yet recognized in DSM-5, nor are the functional consequences of visual–spatial deficits always acknowledged in school settings. Alternatively, students can usually more easily obtain a 504 Plan, which provides individuals with certain accommodations to ensure *access* to education but does not provide modification to the curriculum. Advocates for Children or local special education lawyers can also help guide families to the due process laws in their state. Many services are available to students with disabilities, from speech therapy (ST) to assistive technology (AT) and from classroom accommodations to Special Education Teacher Support Services (SETSS), to name just a few. See Broitman et al. (2020) for a more detailed discussion of these aspects. To our knowledge, Italy is one of the few countries where the definition of provisions for children with special education needs specifically mentions nonverbal learning disability. This inclusive definition has helped in identifying and supporting children with DVSD within schools, without the need to also make reference to other diagnostic categories.
- *Get to know the people who make decisions about your child's education.* This point is strongly related to the previous one. Anyway, having an expert practitioner as a guide could be helpful not only to ask for suggestions but also to manage the complex network around the child's education.
- *Keep records of assessments, meetings, and other educational documents.* As we mentioned before, children with DVSD could receive different diagnoses during their life because this disorder is not well known. Given this situation, it sometimes happens that parents prefer not to share previous diagnoses because they are looking for independent judgments from other practitioners.

In most cases, however, this is not a good idea, as previous documents may help in understanding more clearly the whole picture of the child as well as the developmental trajectory of the disorder.

- *Gather information by reading, attending conferences, and joining support groups.* It is important to keep informed about the main characteristics of the disorder. However, we suggest looking for scientific readings, or experts in the field, and not trusting all information in the web. Not all the information reported in the web and social media is scientifically valid, and it is important to discriminate false from true information, specifically with respect to this profile. Also, support groups and associations of parents may be useful for sharing opinions and experiences. Most parents of children with this disorder feel isolated, and this kind of support may be useful for sharing feelings, emotions, and good-practices. Here (Box 5.1), we will mention some associations in different countries.
- *Communicate effectively, be prepared, and be clear.* This point is strongly related to the previous one. If as a parent, you have understood what DVSD is, you will be able to explain to teachers, other parents, and practitioners the main difficulties of the child in that particular developmental period.
- *Know your child's strengths and interests, and share them with the professionals.* Remember that the strength points of your child are more important than his/her deficits. On the basis of these, important decisions about his or her development may be made.
- *Emphasize solutions.* In discussions with your child, try to suggest ways to solve his/her problems instead of the problem per se. Similarly, ask teachers for solutions to school difficulties, and ask the experts about solutions for solving specific problems.
- *Focus on the big picture.* Although families should be oriented to solve problems that are present in that particular moment, parents may also keep in mind the challenges of dealing with the development of their child, and they need to consider not only the difficulties but also the strength points.
- *Involve your child in decision making as early as it seems reasonable.* Children with DVSD have good intelligence, and they need to be aware of which areas they could and should improve. For this reason, as early as it seems reasonable, it is important to share with them the challenges they have to deal with. The child should be engaged in his/her changes and should be aware of progress during the time course.

- Create a psychologically safe refuge, free from the exhausting demands of the outside world, for your child. Just accomplishing the basic learning activities can be exhausting for these children. Therefore, try to take extra challenges, tasks, or responsibilities off their plate. By removing these things, you are not "enabling them" or preventing them from developing necessary skills. In fact, the opposite is true; you are providing them space to learn and develop at their own pace.
- As a parent, it is critical to actually listen to your child with DVSD and make them feel that you care about their feelings and perceptions of the situation, even if they don't match your own. Develop an open and non-judgmental relationship, which will encourage them to allow you to know what they need help with. This will require checking in with them regarding how things are going. Specifically, ask about their school day and social interactions. Throughout this active listening, the focus should be on trying to solve those issues with your children as *active participants*. Accept that your child's interpretation/perspective is *valid*, and that is the most important issue at stake.
- Finally, as Broitman et al. (2020) point out, help your child to identify triggers that cause stress. A consistent problem is often not knowing your child's boundaries with socialization, academic achievement, etc. Going through each individual issue enables you and your child to be able to plan in advance what may work versus what may be too much.

Box 5.1 Associations of Parents for Nonverbal Learning Disability in the United States, Spain, and Italy

Parents' associations	
United States	The NVLD project www.nvld.org NLD line www.nldline.com/
Spain	Asociación Nacional afectados por el Trastorno de Aprendizaje No Verbal www.tanv.es
Italy	Associazione Italiana per il Disturbo Nonverbale www.aidnv.it

In the next sections, we offer specific suggestions for the most critical areas. In particular, we will consider how to intervene to improve visuospatial and fine-motor skills and socio-relational abilities.

5.2 Tips for Parents to Enhance Visuospatial and Fine-Motor Skills of Their Child

One of the main problems of children with DVSD is dealing with visuospatial information and materials. In Chapter 1, we mentioned that some of these difficulties are struggling with scissors, crayons, or pencils, and generally with drawings, as well as performing fine-motor activities like completing puzzles and playing with construction toys. In order to improve visuospatial abilities with small kids, parents could involve the child in games and video-games that involve visuospatial skills (e.g., Tangram, Lego, or puzzles) or help them shift to more appropriate activities. In Italy, we have published computerized training specifically addressed to parents and teachers, including games that aim to improve visuospatial abilities (Mammarella, Toso, & Caviola, 2011). It is important that children have fun during these activities; hence, parents could guide the child with verbal instruction and could reinforce them positively when the child succeeds. If there are any areas that appear to be of particular interest to the child, it is extremely helpful to support all related activities. We have found that activities that follow the child's passions are most successful. In Box 5.2, we have summarized the main suggestions for parents.

As the child becomes more independent and is able to move around without an adult, parents should offer clear directions and give suggestions about everyday journeys, in particular at the beginning, such as how to reach the gym, how to take the bus, the train, etc. It is useful to accompany them on trial runs to help them anticipate issues and reduce anxiety. Children with DVSD may also have difficulties in reading analog clocks; thus, in this case, parents could shift to using digital clocks. In addition, the child will need help in organizing activities, such as homework, appointments, and plans, but also personal objects that they need to bring back and forth from home and school. Whenever possible, assignments and deadlines should be listed online so that parents can assist with keeping a check on the due date. Parents should help the child by monitoring these activities and in some cases could use images, Post-Its, or written notes, based on the age of the child. Martin (2007), herself the mother of a child with DVSD, acknowledges the burden parents of children with this profile have to create a safe home environment. She stresses the importance of providing a psychologically safe refuge, free from the exhausting demands of the outside world. Just accomplishing the basic learning activities can be exhausting for these children. They will also have a greater need for parental assistance in all areas of life over the course of their lifespan. Parents will need assistance in managing these tasks without fears of infantilizing their children or making them overly dependent. Professionals can and must help parents recognize the appropriateness of parental intervention and involvement (Whitney, 2002).

There are many everyday situations in which our children may need assistance and adaptations, for example, with tying their shoes. In particular, they may encounter difficulties with laces; hence, it could be better to use shoes with Velcro. These are the kinds of simple solutions that can significantly reduce your child's anxiety. Moreover, in acquiring complex motor skills such as riding a tricycle or a bicycle, they will need more time and patience to learn (if they ever do) than the other kids. Overall, for motor skills, parents should adapt the requirements to the level of the child; moreover, verbal prompts will be useful in order to give instructions on what to do. It is important never to forget that verbal skills are these children's strength; hence, a primary aid to the child's learning is to teach them sequentially and to use the child's verbal strengths to compensate whenever possible.

Parents should also pay attention to their child's choice of sporting activities. Some good examples are individual: swimming, judo, karate, or Pilates. Sports in which less competition and social comparison are involved should be generally preferred; team sports are usually less successful, unless otherwise explicitly requested by the child.

Generally speaking, families should balance their wishes to promote their child's independence and the reality that their child requires additional interventions. It is important to maintain a progressive approach, in which parents withdraw support whenever it is no longer needed but are always ready to put it back in if the child encounters something new and novel and cannot quite figure out how to access and generalize previously learned material.

Box 5.2 Main Suggestions That Parents May Use to Promote Visuospatial and Motor Abilities

Visuospatial skills	*Motor abilities*
Introduce and pre-teach games involving visuospatial abilities (e.g., puzzles, Tangram, etc.)	Try to adapt the requirements of motor activities to the level of the child (e.g., shoes with laces)
Encourage your child to draw and paint trying different mediums (e.g., crayons, chalk, finger paints, brush painting, or charcoal)	Pre-teach, expose, and practice games involving motor abilities
Play visuo-constructive activities with your child. For example ask your child to reproduce tridimensional models using blocks and Lego	Encourage fine-motor activities like threading beads onto strings or tying knots and bows in strings
Explicitly describe everyday journeys (e.g., how to take the bus to reach a final destination)	Create games using household items like a small pair of kitchen tongs or tweezers to pick up some small objects like pasta or buttons and transfer them into a bowl
Use digital clocks instead of analog ones	Encourage your child in using scissors to improve hand–eye coordination (e.g., cutting around drawn shapes, cutting play-dough)
Schedule the time for managing concrete activities	Carefully choose sport/team activities

5.3 Tips for Parents to Deal with Social Skills Problems of Children with DVSD

Brett said:

> I experienced difficulty with an unbelievably large set of activities, but I had one where I excelled, and that was speaking. I could talk up a storm, and that ability set up a long-lasting confusion in my life—why did adults (who weren't my teachers) connect so easily to me, while kids didn't seem to like me

> at all? I know that this is probably something that a lot of kids have asked themselves, but my version of the question seemed very profound to me at the time; I felt like I was two different people. I did not make an active choice to act differently, but the difference in my experience with my peers versus my experience with my parents and their friends was so extreme that it felt like I was living in two different realities. At school I felt lost and confused. I had no friends, and was either picked on or ignored. In class I was trying hard to keep my head down and get out as quickly as humanly possible. At home and around other adults I believe that my social ineptitudes were apparent, but I was not aware of this at the time.
>
> (Broitman & Davis, 2013, p. 330)

In the preceding paragraph, Brett explains one of the main problems of children with DVSD, which is peer social relationships. Often, these children feel easier in interactions with adults than with peers. In peer relations, children with DVSD may encounter social difficulties, such as in interpreting facial expressions as well as in nonverbal communication and socializing. They may have difficulties in understanding irony and jokes, and their poor motor issues might reduce their interaction with peers, exacerbating the problems.

The child could need training in social skills and pragmatics. In clinical practice, this is sometimes done in groups, and finding these types of groups may be difficult, but as understanding of DVSD increases, so do the resources. These groups can be led by private clinicians or psychologists or in general, by expert practitioners. However, we have often found that our children with DVSD do better in one-on-one work. Families may also be very helpful in improving the social skills of their child. A child's social isolation and dependency on parents may be a typical family problem.

Parents may need help in understanding how to positively approach promoting an active self-help role for their child. They can use direct instruction to teach their child how to develop and refine the social skills necessary for meaningful social relationships and interactions with peers. Through modeling (e.g., providing visual examples of how to do something), verbal reinforcements (e.g., good job, great ...), creation of useful opportunities, and providing direct instruction, parents may help the child to progress socially. External positive reinforcements, such as rewards, are sometimes necessary. When the child manifests appropriate social skills during everyday life, immediate encouragement should be tied to the performance. It is also important for the child to perceive the social interaction as meaningful, so parents should explicitly explain why it is important. Appropriate reinforcement may also promote peer engagement and more importantly, may maintain the child's motivation to interact with other people. It may be useful for the child with DVSD to practice social interaction followed by reflection on the mental states of himself or herself and the others in the interaction. Movies and performance-based games supporting the imitation of facial expressions and social role-playing may be similarly helpful, along with verbalizing or journaling to foster reflection and utilize the verbal processing of these activities. A co-created journal could include pictures, emotions, a list of situations encountered, dialog, and the reflections of the child about the experience. If the child is interested, a drama course may be suggested. Drama and acting have often been a successful avenue for our children. Children with DVSD may have difficulties in accurately perceiving and integrating nonverbal cues in social interactions, such as facial expressions, voice intonations, and gestures. Such deficits may results in inappropriate behaviors and the inability to build and maintain satisfactory relationships. Watching movies or TV together is an excellent opportunity to talk through social interactions. Parents can verbalize the feelings and emotions of the actors, and then, they could ask to the child to do the same (see a summary of suggestions in Box 5.3).

5.4 Tips for Parents to Deal with School Difficulties

In the last chapter, we have proposed a series of suggestions for teachers or educators who work with children with DVSD. Here, briefly, we will summarize how parents could help children with DVSD deal with school difficulties. As previously mentioned, these children often develop early math difficulties, such as in discriminating or estimating quantity. During primary school, symptoms might emerge more clearly, and difficulties in handwriting, conceptual mathematics, geometry, and math-based science may become manifest. It should be noted that school difficulties will result from their visuospatial processing deficits, with a variety of differences among children, which can change over the course of their development. In other words, school problems are not derived from specific

Box 5.3 Main Suggestions That Parents May Use to Promote Social Skills

Social skills
Give direct instructions to the child about what to do in social situations
Verbally explain how to use a nonverbal cues or facial expressions to infer a particular emotion
Discuss with your child what are appropriate or inappropriate behaviors during social exchanges
Watch movies and discuss with the child the emotions expressed by the actors.
Create games with drama of social relations, and watch brief part of movies without audio for focusing on nonverbal cues
Suggest to the child how to ask for more explanation if something in a social exchange is not clear
Promote safe supervised after-school activities with peers
Invite the friends of your child at home for play dates

learning disorders (rather, in some cases, a specific learning disorder may be present as a comorbidity) and for this reason, could change according to the characteristics of the child. Teachers and expert practitioners may work on specific deficits by suggesting individualized educational plans or specific interventions. Parents should pay attention to improvements or difficulties encountered in doing homework and should signal to teachers if a specific task is too difficult for the child, requesting modifications when needed. Parents can also help the child to create a realistic schedule for doing their different activities and exercises at home, and should establish routines, such as the space of the house dedicated to studying and the time for doing homework, being sure to build in the breaks and pauses necessary between one activity and another.

If school is limited to the morning hours, as may happen in some countries, homework and afternoon activities can be supervised by a tutor who supports the child, avoiding a conflict-prone interaction between the parent and child over homework. However, if parents prefer to help the child, they should be mindful of the complexities of working with their child. Specific attention should be devoted to tasks and activities that require great involvement of visuospatial and fine-motor abilities (e.g., mathematics, geometry, handwriting, drawing, etc.). If the child is not able to perform a particular assignment, parents should communicate with teachers and request modifications or accommodations as needed. Finally, the engagement and motivation of the child to perform difficult tasks should be reinforced by the parents. It is important to recognize the effort and the dedication required for the child to perform school activities (see a summary of these suggestions in Box 5.4).

Box 5.4 Main Suggestions That Parents May Use to Promote School Activities

School activities
Maintain continuous exchange with teachers and expert practitioners who know the child and signal when an activity is too difficult to perform.
To avoid conflict with your child, and if possible, ask for a tutor who can supervise your child in school activities. If you prefer to supervise your child, try always promoting their autonomy providing help only when it is needed
If possible, did not replace an activity assigned to your child but try to implement modifications in order to adapt the activity to the child abilities
Reinforce motivation and dedication to school activities and success in performing difficult tasks

5.5 How to Cope with Parenting Stress and Help Your Child

Parenting stress is an important variable to consider when providing intervention to families with children with DVSD (McDowell, Saylor, Taylor, Boyce, & Stokes, 1995). Parental stress is associated with increased maternal depression (Lipman, Boyle, Dooley, & Offord, 2002; Margalit, Raviv, & Ankonina, 1992). It is clear that high levels of stress and/or depression interfere with parenting (Webster-Stratton, 1990). We have learned that several variables have been found to influence parenting stress. Socioeconomic status is inversely related to levels of parenting stress (Kazdin, Stolar, & Marciano, 1995), meaning that parental stress increases when socioeconomic status is low. This intuitively makes sense, as when resources are limited, it can be harder to get outside tutors and help. High levels of stress have been observed in parents (Tunali & Power, 1993; Antshel & Joseph, 2006). In particular, some findings seem to suggest that single-parent households appear more likely to report higher levels of parenting stress (Thompson, Auslander, & Whit, 2001) when children are developmentally disabled in some way. Not surprisingly, boys are perceived as more stressful than girls, and older children are perceived as more stressful for parents. Again, this confirms that it takes a lot of effort and energy to raise children with DVSD.

However, it is extremely important to note that there is evidence that the stress experienced by the parent decreases with effective treatment, even when parental stress is not the focus of the intervention (Kazdin & Wassell, 2000). Families can be supported and advised in a series of problems they may meet with children with DVSD or that children may present within the family context. Based on different reports, Davis and Broitman (2011) mention a series of health risks of which parents should be aware. They mention, for example, the risk of injuries related to poor attention and motor coordination and the risk of weight increase due to a sedentary life. Hence, according to Davis and Broitman (2011), child variables within the family context must also be considered when suggesting interventions for families involving children with DVSD.

Although training programs designed specifically for parents of children with DVSD are not available, there are good reasons for expecting that parent training could be as useful as it has been for other clinical groups. In particular, support programs for parents of children with similar symptoms, such as attention-deficit hyperactivity disorder (ADHD), autism spectrum disorders, or specific learning disorders, are likely to benefit parents of children with DVSD (see for example, Chronis, Chacko, Fabiano, Wymbs, & Pelham, 2004). Some of the common themes in parent training include basic psychoeducation on neurodevelopmental disorders, how to recognize critical issues, coping strategies, increasing consistency and authoritative parenting practices, coping with educational issues, and sharing family problems with other families who have similar situations.

As a parent, you may consider these simple and general suggestions. First, the most important thing you can do for your child is to actually listen to them and make them feel that you care about their feelings and perceptions of the situation, even if they do not match your own. Throughout active listening, the focus should be on trying to solve some issues with your children as active participants—that means finding solutions that actually solve the problem for them rather than what would work for you, or fit a specific diagnosis, or be easiest (Broitman et al., 2020).

Second, you should accept that your child already knows that they are different in some way, whether or not they have received or have been told about an official diagnosis. While your feelings around a diagnosis may involve worries about labels and inevitable limitations, know that for your child, thinking there is "something unknown and wrong with them" is infinitely worse. In fact, having a diagnosis means that your child is now exposed to the idea that there are other people like them out there, which is much more hopeful than thinking they are literally alone. Processing what it means to have a diagnosis and intervention is difficult for the whole family, not just the individual with DVSD. This process is likely to be at least somewhat painful and guilt-inducing for parents (and at times the siblings), as they come to better understand the challenges and pain the child is going through. The family will have to accept that there is a limited extent to which their pain and guilt can help alleviate their child's pain (Broitman et al., 2020).

Another area of support you can provide for your child is to help them develop processes. A lot of where your child's energy gets used up every day is often in attempting to accomplish tasks that you, as a neurotypical, may find incredibly easy. Best not to start saying "don't worry, this will be easy" (Broitman et al., 2020). Helping your child identify weak points and then, crucially, building simple and straightforward processes to cope/compensate can help give them confidence and skills going forward (Tsatsanis and Rourke, 2003). An expert practitioner will often also work on these sorts of skills, especially in academic settings, but the need for processes like this also applies to non-academic settings, which are a great way for you to get directly involved, if you and your child want that level of involvement.

In addition, parents should help the child identify triggers that cause stress or anxiety: likely a consistent problem underlying other weak areas is not knowing where your child's boundaries are with socialization. Going through each individual area and trying to talk through boundaries enables you and your child to be able to plan in advance what may work versus what may be too much (Broitman et al., 2020).

As a final suggestion, the most important in our opinion, parents should enjoy the time spent with their child and not think of every difficulty as a function of the disorder. Every child is different from every other, and every child may encounter difficulties in his/her life. Children with DVSD need to be recognized for their strengths and not only for their difficulties. We would like to conclude this chapter with the words of the mother of a child with DVSD.

> When I look at his current success, I have great awe and admiration for his perseverance and strength. Brett is an independent, professional young man with clear goals and a realistic plan for obtaining them. He has talent, passion, and healthy close relationships. He knows how to use his unique and creative mind. Life truly got better for Brett once he was out of middle school! One of the secrets to his success was that we were able to pull together and thoroughly use a superb team of professionals. They made it their mission and business to figure out what Brett needed to successfully learn. My model was that if he didn't understand me, it was my error and I needed to learn how to explain it better so that he could understand.
>
> (Broitman & Davis, 2013, p. 346)

Conclusions

In this book, we have offered our knowledge and our experience in order to help parents and teachers in promoting best practices for optimizing the development of their children with nonverbal learning disability, or as we are now referring to it, developmental visuospatial disorder (DVSD). As we have reported, this disorder is less understood than other learning disabilities, and confusion remains over differentiating it from other somewhat similar neurodevelopmental disorders. In this book we provided a thorough description of this clinical condition and integrated the most recent results from the world of scientific research with the most relevant knowledge from clinical and educational practice. Our goal is to support parents and teachers to help children with DVSD to achieve their potential. We believe this knowledge will allow them to tailor their interventions at home, in the classroom, and in a social context. Our hope is that this book has shed more light on both the main strengths and the difficulties these children could encounter in their life. We strongly believe that children with DVSD can succeed in their life and find their way to achieving their goals by using their strengths. Of course, we recognize that this can be a daunting task, as they will encounter many challenges during their life. However, they can be helped to cope with those difficulties at school as well as during social interactions. Teachers and parents can support their development; the most important lesson we think you can give them is to believe in their own abilities and in their potential to cope with challenges. There is no one right way to teach these skills. Parents may help them learn how to listen to their needs, how to advocate for themselves, and how to protect them from becoming overwhelmed by having a neurodevelopmental disorder. They can instill in them trust and respect for themselves. Moreover, they can teach them to think about what kind of life will work best for them. Alongside parents, teachers can support these students by providing clear and realistic expectations and learning goals tailored to the specific characteristics of the student's profile. They may also present challenging but attainable tasks divided into manageable chunks when this is needed (i.e., when the tasks include visuospatial demands) and constructive feedback and explanations. In addition, parents and teachers can help children with DVSD by facilitating their social inclusion and supporting them from an emotional and motivational point of view.

Another aim of our book was to summarize the main suggestions we derived from our experience with children with DVSD. We believe that our general recommendations could be useful to teachers and parents in dealing with the challenges they have to face in everyday life. It is worth noting that our suggestions are not tailored to the characteristics of a specific child; hence, they might not always be appropriate, since although children with DVSD generally share some deficits and strengths, every child with DVSD is unique, as is every one of us. It is for this reason that we have highlighted the need to have the assistance of an expert practitioner or a team of experts. Those experts could give more specific suggestions, as they have met your child personally and know what your child really needs. In other words, parents and teachers should take inspiration from our general suggestions, which, at the same time, need to be personalized for each specific case.

In this regard, we would now like to tell you something about the children we cited in the first chapters of our book: Fabrizio and Alex. Fabrizio is now 11 years old. We have followed his progress for 2 years, and after a brief intervention to improve his handwriting, we have worked with him and a small group on social skills in order to enhance his self-confidence and to give him more strategies to interact properly with peers. With his parents, he decided to start attending boy scout groups, where he established new friendships. We have worked with teachers, suggesting to them the best ways to help Fabrizio at school, and at the moment, it seems successful. Of course, there will be new challenges when he reaches preadolescence, and we are ready to discuss possible next steps with Fabrizio and his family in order to support them along his development path.

What about Alex? He has already found his favorite hobby, which is rowing. During the intervention, we worked with teachers on his math difficulties. Teachers are helping him, but he is still having troubles with math. However, he has started an acting course to gain self-confidence, and he is happy because he can talk with people with similar interests. An area in which he is encountering difficulties now is in his relations with his parents. He is trying to becoming more independent, but at the same time, he still needs them, and this is causing conflicts at the moment. His parents have asked us for some suggestions in order to deal with this situation. These examples show how children with DVSD are different and in what sense they need tailored interventions, based on their age of development, their characteristics, and their feelings.

To conclude this book, we would like to remind parents that the most important thing they can do for their child is actually listen to them and make the child feel that they care about their feelings and perceptions of the situation. Listen to your child, focus on trying to figure out where they are in pain, and discuss with them possible concrete solutions for the problem. It is important to recognize, however, that during adolescence, one wants to respect their need to become more independent, Parents should continue to be actively present and offer help when asked. We would also like to remind teachers that they, too, play a crucial role in the development of children with DVSD. They can contribute positively to the development of self-esteem and sense of self-efficacy of these students by supporting them from both an academic and a social perspective. Hopefully, you will share our optimism that children with DVSD can successfully face the challenges ahead.

References

Allen, G. L., Kirasic, K. C., Dobson, S. H., Long, R. G., & Beck, S. (1996). Predicting environmental learning from spatial abilities: An indirect route. *Intelligence*, *22*(3), 327–355.

Alloway, T. P., & Archibald, L. (2008). Working memory and learning in children with developmental coordination disorder and specific language impairment. *Journal of Learning Disabilities*, *41*(3), 251–262.

American Psychiatric Association. (2000). *Diagnostic criteria from DSM-IV-TR*. American Psychiatric Publishing.

American Psychiatric Association. (2013). *Diagnostic and statistical manual of mental disorders (DSM-5®)*. Washington, DC: American Psychiatric Publishing.

Antshel, K. M., & Joseph, G. R. (2006). Maternal stress in nonverbal learning disorder: A comparison with reading disorder. *Journal of Learning Disabilities*, *39*(3), 194–205.

Bachot, J., Gevers, W., Fias, W., & Roeyers, H. (2005). Number sense in children with visuospatial disabilities: Orientation of the mental number line. *Psychology Science*, *47*(1), 172.

Banker, S. M., Ramphal, B., Pagliaccio, D., et al. (2020a). Spatial network connectivity and spatial reasoning ability in children with nonverbal learning disability. *Scientific Reports*, *10*, 561. doi: 10.1038/s41598-019-56003-y

Banker, S. M., Pagliaccio, D., Ramphal, B., Thomas, L., Dranovsky, A., & Margolis, A. E. (2020b). Altered structure and functional connectivity of the hippocampus are associated with social and mathematical difficulties in nonverbal learning disability. *Hippocampus*, 1–10. doi: 10.1002/hipo.23264

Benton, A. L., Hamsher, K., Varney, N. R., & Spreen, O. (1983). *Contributions to neuropsychological assessment. A clinical manual.* New York: Oxford University Press.

Bloom, E., & Heath, N. (2010). Recognition, expression, and understanding facial expressions of emotion in adolescents with nonverbal and general learning disabilities. *Journal of Learning Disabilities*, *43*(2), 180–192.

Broitman, J., & Davis, J. (2013). *Treating NVLD children*. New York: Springer.

Broitman, J., Melcher, M., Margolis, A., & Davis, J. M. (2020). *NVLD and developmental visual-spatial disorder in children*. Cham: Springer.

Brumback, R. A. (1985). Neurology of depression. *Neurology and Neurosurgery Update Series*, *7*(6), 1–8.

Bühler, E., Bachmann, C., Goyert, H., Heinzel-Gutenbrunner, M., & Kamp-Becker, I. (2011). Differential diagnosis of autism spectrum disorder and attention deficit hyperactivity disorder by means of inhibitory control and 'theory of mind'. *Journal of Autism and Developmental Disorders*, *41*(12), 1718–1726.

Capodieci, A., Crisci, G., & Mammarella, I. C. (2019). Does positive illusory bias affect self-concept and loneliness in children with symptoms of ADHD? *Journal of Attention Disorders*, *23*(11), 1274–1283.

Cardillo, R., Garcia, R. B., Mammarella, I. C., & Cornoldi, C. (2018). Pragmatics of language and theory of mind in children with dyslexia with associated language difficulties or nonverbal learning disabilities. *Applied Neuropsychology: Child*, *7*(3), 245–256.

Cardillo, R., Vio, C., & Mammarella, I. C. (2020). A comparison of local-global visuospatial processing in autism spectrum disorder, nonverbal learning disability, ADHD and typical development. *Research in Developmental Disabilities*, *103*, 103682.

Carpenter Rich, E., Loo, S. K., Yang, M., Dang, J., & Smalley, S. L. (2009). Social functioning difficulties in ADHD: Association with PDD risk. *Clinical Child Psychology and Psychiatry*, *14*(3), 329–344.

Chow, D., & Skuy, M. (1999). Simultaneous and successive cognitive processing in children with nonverbal learning disabilities. *School Psychology International*, *20*(2), 219–231.

Chronis, A. M., Chacko, A., Fabiano, G. A., Wymbs, B. T., & Pelham, W. E. (2004). Enhancements to the behavioral parent training paradigm for families of children with ADHD: Review and future directions. *Clinical Child and Family Psychology Review*, *7*(1), 1–27.

Collins, A., Brown, J. S., & Newman, S. E. (1988). Cognitive apprenticeship: Teaching the craft of reading, writing and mathematics. *Thinking: The Journal of Philosophy for Children*, *8*(1), 2–10.

Cornoldi, C. (1997). *Abilità visuo-spaziali: intervento sulle difficoltà non verbali di apprendimento* (Vol. 51). Edizioni Erickson.

Cornoldi, C., Mammarella, I. C., & Fine, J. G. (2016). *Nonverbal learning disabilities*. Guilford Press.

Cornoldi, C., Rigoni, F., Tressoldi, P. E., & Vio, C. (1999). Imagery deficits in nonverbal learning disabilities. *Journal of Learning Disabilities*, *32*(1), 48–57.

Cornoldi, C., Vecchia, R. D., & Tressoldi, P. E. (1995). Visuo-spatial working memory limitations in low visuo-spatial high verbal intelligence children. *Journal of Child Psychology and Psychiatry*, *36*(6), 1053–1064.

Cornoldi, C., Venneri, A., Marconato, F., Molin, A., & Montinari, C. (2003). A rapid screening measure for the identification of visuospatial learning disability in schools. *Journal of Learning Disabilities*, *36*(4), 299–306.

Crollen, V., Vanderclausen, C., Allaire, F., Pollaris, A., & Noël, M. P. (2016). Spatial and numerical processing in children with non-verbal learning disabilities. *Research in Developmental Disabilities*, *47*, 61–72.

Davis, J. M., & Broitman, J. (2011). *Nonverbal learning disabilities in children: Bridging the gap between science and practice*. Springer Science+Business Media.

Delis, D. C., Kaplan, E., & Kramer, J. H. (2001). *Delis-Kaplan executive function system (D- KEFS)*. London, UK: Psychological Corporation.

Denis, M., Daniel, M. P., Fontaine, S., & Pazzaglia, F. (2001). Language, spatial cognition, and navigation. *Imagery, Language and Visuo-Spatial Thinking*, 137–160.

Dimitrovsky, L., Spector, H., Levy-Shiff, R., & Vakil, E. (1998). Interpretation of facial expressions of affect in children with learning disabilities with verbal or nonverbal deficits. *Journal of Learning Disabilities*, *31*(3), 286–292.

Drummond, C. R., Ahmad, S. A., & Rourke, B. P. (2005). Rules for the classification of younger children with nonverbal learning disabilities and basic phonological processing disabilities. *Archives of Clinical Neuropsychology*, *20*(2), 171–182.

Durand, M. (2005). Is there a fine motor skill deficit in nonverbal learning disabilities. *Educational & Child Psychology*, 22, 90–99.

Ferrara, R., & Mammarella, I. C. (2013). Il Questionario SVS Bambino. *Psicologia Clinica dello Sviluppo*, *17*(2), 359–0.

Fine, J. G., Musielak, K. A., & Semrud-Clikeman, M. (2014). Smaller splenium in children with nonverbal learning disability compared to controls, high-functioning autism and ADHD. *Child Neuropsychology*, *20*(6), 641–661.

Fisher, N. J., Deluca, J. W., & Rourke, B. P. (1997). Wisconsin Card Sorting Test and Halstead Category Test performances of children and adolescents who exhibit the syndrome of nonverbal learning disabilities. *Child Neuropsychology*, *3*(1), 61–70.

Fletcher, J. M. (1985). External validation of learning disability typologies. In B. P. Rourke (Ed.), *Neuropsychology of learning disabilities: Essentials of subtype analysis* (pp. 187–211). The Guilford Press.

Forrest, B. J. (2004). The utility of math difficulties, internalized psychopathology, and visual-spatial deficits to identify children with the nonverbal learning disability syndrome: Evidence for a visualspatial disability. *Child Neuropsychology*, *10*(2), 129–146.

Foss, J. M. (1991). Nonverbal learning disabilities and remedial interventions. *Annals of Dyslexia*, *41*(1), 128–140.

Fournier, K. A., Hass, C. J., Naik, S. K., Lodha, N., & Cauraugh, J. H. (2010). Motor coordination in autism spectrum disorders: A synthesis and meta-analysis. *Journal of Autism and Developmental Disorders*, *40*(10), 1227–1240.

Frith, U. (1989). A new look at language and communication in autism. *International Journal of Language & Communication Disorders*, *24*(2), 123–150.

Garcia, R. B., Mammarella, I. C., Tripodi, D., & Cornoldi, C. (2014). Visuospatial working memory for locations, colours, and binding in typically developing children and in children with dyslexia and non-verbal learning disability. *British Journal of Developmental Psychology*, *32*(1), 17–33.

Gerstmann, J. (1940). Syndrome of finger agnosia, disorientation for right and left, agraphia and acalculia: Local diagnostic value. *Archives of Neurology & Psychiatry*, *44*(2), 398–408.

Gillberg, C. (2003). Deficits in attention, motor control, and perception: A brief review. *Archives of Disease in Childhood*, *88*(10), 904–910.

Gillberg, C., Winnegar, I., & Gillberg, C. (1993). Screening methods, epidemiology, and evaluation of intervention in DAMP in preschool children. *European Child and Adolescent Psychiatry*, 2, 121–135.

Goodwin, M. W. (1999). Cooperative learning and social skills: What skills to teach and how to teach them. *Intervention in School and Clinic*, *35*(1), 29–33.

Griffin, J. R., & Grisham, J. D. (2002). *Binocular anomalies: Diagnosis and vision therapy*. Butterworth-Heinemann Medical.

Guillot, A., Hoyek, N., Louis, M., & Collet, C. (2012). Understanding the timing of motor imagery: Recent findings and future directions. *International Review of Sport and Exercise Psychology*, *5*(1), 3–22.

Hale, J. B., & Fiorello, C. A. (2004). *School neuropsychology*. New York: Guilford.

Harnadek, M. C., & Rourke, B. P. (1994). Principal identifying features of the syndrome of nonverbal learning disabilities in children. *Journal of Learning Disabilities*, *27*(3), 144–154.

Hegarty, M., Montello, D. R., Richardson, A. E., Ishikawa, T., & Lovelace, K. (2006). Spatial abilities at different scales: Individual differences in aptitude-test performance and spatial-layout learning. *Intelligence*, *34*(2), 151–176.

Heiman, T. (2005). An examination of peer relationships of children with and without attention deficit hyperactivity disorder. *School Psychology International*, *26*(3), 330–339.

Hodgens, J. B., Cole, J., & Boldizar, J. (2000). Peer-based differences among boys with ADHD. *Journal of Clinical Child Psychology*, *29*(3), 443–452.

Hoza, B., Mrug, S., Gerdes, A. C., Hinshaw, S. P., Bukowski, W. M., Gold, J. A.,... & Arnold, L. E. (2005). What aspects of peer relationships are impaired in children with attention-deficit/hyperactivity disorder? *Journal of Consulting and Clinical Psychology*, *73*(3), 411.

Hubbard, E. M., Piazza, M., Pinel, P., & Dehaene, S. (2005). Interactions between number and space in parietal cortex. *Nature Reviews. Neuroscience*, *6*(6), 435–448.

Humphries, T., Cardy, J. O., Worling, D. E., & Peets, K. (2004). Narrative comprehension and retelling abilities of children with nonverbal learning disabilities. *Brain and Cognition*, *56*(1), 77–88.

Inhelder, B., & Piaget, J. (1964). *The early growth of logic in the child*, trans. E. A. Lunzer and D. Papert.

Jansen, P., & Lehmann, J. (2013). Mental rotation performance in soccer players and gymnasts in an object-based mental rotation task. *Advances in Cognitive Psychology*, *9*(2), 92.

Jarrett, M. A., & Ollendick, T. H. (2008). A conceptual review of the comorbidity of attention-deficit/hyperactivity disorder and anxiety: Implications for future research and practice. *Clinical Psychology Review*, *28*(7), 1266–1280.

Johnson, D. J., & Myklebust, H. R. (1967). *Learning disabilities; educational principles and practices*. New York: Grune & Stratton, 367.

Johnson-Laird, P. N. (1983). *Mental models: Towards a cognitive science of language, inference, and consciousness (No. 6)*. Harvard University Press.

Jordan, D. W., & Métais, J. L. (1997). Social skilling through cooperative learning. *Educational Research*, *39*(1), 3–21.

Kadzin, A. E., Stolar, M. J., & Marciano, P. L. (1995). Risk factors for dropping out of treatment among White and Black families. *Journal of Family Psychology*, *9*(4), 402.

Kazdin, A. E., & Wassell, G. (2000). Therapeutic changes in children, parents, and families resulting from treatment of children with conduct problems. *Journal of the American Academy of Child & Adolescent Psychiatry*, *39*(4), 414–420.

Khouzam, H. R., El-Gabalawi, F., Pirwani, N., & Priest, F. (2004). Asperger's disorder: A review of its diagnosis and treatment. *Comprehensive Psychiatry*, *45*(3), 184–191.

Klin, A., Volkmar, F. R., & Sparrow, S. S. (Eds.). (2000). *Asperger syndrome* (pp. 1–21). New York: Guilford Press.

Klin, A., Volkmar, F. R., Sparrow, S. S., Cicchetti, D. V., & Rourke, B. P. (1995). Validity and neuropsychological characterization of Asperger syndrome: Convergence with nonverbal learning disabilities syndrome. *Journal of Child Psychology and Psychiatry*, *36*(7), 1127–1140.

Korkman, M., Kemp, S. L., & Kirk, U. (2001). Developmental assessment of neuropsychological function with the aid. In A. S. Kaufman, & N. M. Kaufman. *Specific learning disabilities and difficulties in children and adolescents: Psychological assessment and evaluation*. Cambridge University Press, Cambridge, UK.

Kozhevnikov, M., Motes, M. A., Rasch, B., & Blajenkova, O. (2006). Perspective-taking vs. mental rotation transformations and how they predict spatial navigation performance. *Applied Cognitive Psychology: The Official Journal of the Society for Applied Research in Memory and Cognition*, *20*(3), 397–417.

Labate, E., Pazzaglia, F., & Hegarty, M. (2014). What working memory subcomponents are needed in the acquisition of survey knowledge? Evidence from direction estimation and shortcut tasks. *Journal of Environmental Psychology*, *37*, 73–79.

Lavoie, R. (1994). Do's & don'ts for fostering social competence. Retrieved on November, 6, 2000.

Lipman, E. L., Boyle, M. H., Dooley, M. D., & Offord, D. R. (2002). Child well-being in single-mother families. *Journal of the American Academy of Child & Adolescent Psychiatry*, *41*(1), 75–82.

Magill-Evans, J., Koning, C., Cameron-Sadava, A., & Manyk, K. (1995). The child and adolescent social perception measure. *Journal of Nonverbal Behavior*, *19*(3), 151–169.

Mammarella, I. C., Bomba, M., Caviola, S., Broggi, F., Neri, F., Lucangeli, D., & Nacinovich, R. (2013). Mathematical difficulties in nonverbal learning disability or co-morbid dyscalculia and dyslexia. *Developmental Neuropsychology*, *38*(6), 418–432.

Mammarella, I. C., Cardillo, R., & Zoccante, L. (2019). Differences in visuospatial processing in individuals with nonverbal learning disability or autism spectrum disorder without intellectual disability. *Neuropsychology*, *33*(1), 123.

Mammarella, I. C., & Cornoldi, C. (2005a). Difficulties in the control of irrelevant visuospatial information in children with visuospatial learning disabilities. *Acta Psychologica*, *118*(3), 211–228.

Mammarella, I. C., & Cornoldi, C. (2005b). Sequence and space: The critical role of a backward spatial span in the working memory deficit of visuospatial learning disabled children. *Cognitive Neuropsychology*, *22*(8), 1055–1068.

Mammarella, I. C., & Cornoldi, C. (2014). An analysis of the criteria used to diagnose children with Nonverbal Learning Disability (NLD). *Child Neuropsychology*, *20*(3), 255–280.

Mammarella, I. C., & Cornoldi, C. (2019). Nonverbal learning disability (developmental visuospatial disorder), in A. Gallagher, C. Bulteau-Peyrie,

D. Cohen, & J. Michaud (Eds.), *Neurocognitive development: Part II disorders and disabilities*. Academic Press, Elsevier.

Mammarella, I. C., Cornoldi, C., Pazzaglia, F., Toso, C., Grimoldi, M., & Vio, C. (2006). Evidence for a double dissociation between spatial-simultaneous and spatial-sequential working memory in visuospatial (nonverbal) learning disabled children. *Brain and Cognition*, *62*(1), 58–67.

Mammarella, I. C., Ghisi, M., Bomba, M., Bottesi, G., Caviola, S., Broggi, F., & Nacinovich, R. (2016). Anxiety and depression in children with nonverbal learning disabilities, reading disabilities, or typical development. *Journal of Learning Disabilities*, *49*(2), 130–139.

Mammarella, I. C., Giofrè, D., Ferrara, R., & Cornoldi, C. (2013). Intuitive geometry and visuospatial working memory in children showing symptoms of nonverbal learning disabilities. *Child Neuropsychology*, *19*(3), 235–249.

Mammarella, I. C., & Lipparini, S. (2015). Un intervento sulla comprensione del testo e sul metodo di studio in un caso di disturbo dell'apprendimento non verbale. *Psicologia Clinica dello Sviluppo*, *19*(1), 165–176.

Mammarella, I. C., Lucangeli, D., & Cornoldi, C. (2010). Spatial working memory and arithmetic deficits in children with nonverbal learning difficulties. *Journal of Learning Disabilities*, *43*(5), 455–468.

Mammarella, I. C., Meneghetti, C., Pazzaglia, F., & Cornoldi, C. (2015). Memory and comprehension deficits in spatial descriptions of children with non-verbal and reading disabilities. *Frontiers in Psychology*, *5*, 1534.

Mammarella, I. C., Meneghetti, C., Pazzaglia, F., Gitti, F., Gomez, C., & Cornoldi, C. (2009). Representation of survey and route spatial descriptions in children with nonverbal (visuospatial) learning disabilities. *Brain and Cognition*, *71*(2), 173–179.

Mammarella, I. C., & Pazzaglia, F. (2010). Visual perception and memory impairments in children at risk of nonverbal learning disabilities. *Child Neuropsychology*, *16*(6), 564–576.

Mammarella, I. C., Toso, C., & Caviola, S. (2011). *Che memoria... spaziale!* [Which memory...spatial!]. Trento: Erisckon

Margalit, M., Raviv, A., & Ankonina, D. B. (1992). Coping and coherence among parents with disabled children. *Journal of Clinical Child and Adolescent Psychology*, *21*(3), 202–209.

Margolis, A. E., Broitman, J., Davis, J. M., Alexander, L., Hamilton, A., Liao, Z., ... & Merikangas, K. (2020). Estimated prevalence of nonverbal learning disability among North American children and adolescents. *JAMA Network Open*, *3*(4), e202551–e202551.

Margolis, A. E., Pagliaccio, D., Thomas, L., Banker, S., & Marsh, R. (2019). Salience network connectivity and social processing in children with nonverbal learning disability or autism spectrum disorder. *Neuropsychology*, *33*(1), 135–143.

Martin, M. (2007). *Helping children with nonverbal learning disabilities to flourish: A guide for parents and professionals*. Jessica Kingsley Publishers.

Martinussen, R., Hayden, J., Hogg-Johnson, S., & Tannock, R. (2005). A meta-analysis of working memory impairments in children with attention-deficit/hyperactivity disorder. *Journal of the American Academy of Child & Adolescent Psychiatry*, *44*(4), 377–384.

Matte, R. R., & Bolaski, J. A. (1998). Nonverbal learning disabilities: An overview. *Intervention in School and Clinic*, *34*(1), 39–42.

McDowell, A. D., Saylor, C. F., Taylor, M. J., Boyce, G. C., & Stokes, S. J. (1995). Ethnicity and parenting stress change during early intervention. *Early Child Development and Care*, *111*(1), 131–140.

Mokros, H. B., Poznanski, E. O., & Merrick, W. A. (1989). Depression and learning disabilities in children: A test of an hypothesis. *Journal of Learning Disabilities*, *22*(4), 230–233.

Molenaar-Klumper, M. (2002). *Nonverbal learning disabilities*. London: Jessica Kingsley Publishers.

Mrug, S., Hoza, B., Pelham, W. E., Gnagy, E. M., & Greiner, A. R. (2007). Behavior and peer status in children with ADHD: Continuity and change. *Journal of Attention Disorders*, *10*(4), 359–371.

Münzer, S., Fehringer, B. C., & Kühl, T. (2018). Specificity of mental transformations involved in understanding spatial structures. *Learning and Individual Differences*, *61*, 40–50.

Murray, M. J. (2010). Attention-deficit/hyperactivity disorder in the context of autism spectrum disorders. *Current Psychiatry Reports*, *12*(5), 382–388.

Nichelli, P., & Venneri, A. (1995). Right hemisphere developmental learning disability: A case study. *Neurocase*, *1*(2), 173–177.

Nydén, A., Niklasson, L., Ståhlberg, O., Anckarsäter, H., Dahlgren-Sandberg, A., Wentz, E., & Råstam, M. (2010). Adults with Asperger syndrome with and without a cognitive profile associated with "non-verbal learning disability." A brief report. *Research in Autism Spectrum Disorders*, *4*(4), 612–618.

Osmon, D. C., Smerz, J. M., Braun, M. M., & Plambeck, E. (2006). Processing abilities associated with math skills in adult learning disability. *Journal of Clinical and Experimental Neuropsychology*, *28*(1), 84–95.

Palombo, J., & Berenberg, A. H. (1999). Working with parents of children with nonverbal learning disabilities: A conceptual and intervention model. *Understanding, diagnosing, and treating AD/HD in children and adolescents: An integrated approach*, 389–441.

Pazzaglia, F., & De Beni, R. (2006). Are people with high and low mental rotation abilities differently susceptible to the alignment effect? *Perception*, *35*(3), 369–383.

Pearson, A., Ropar, D., & Hamilton, A. F. D. (2013). A review of visual perspective taking in autism spectrum disorder. *Frontiers in Human Neuroscience*, *7*, 652.

Pennington, B. F. (1991). Right hemisphere learning disorders. *Diagnosing learning disorders: A neuropsychological framework*, 111–134.

Pennington, B. F. (2009). Nonverbal learning disability. *Diagnosing learning disorders: A neuropsychological framework*, 242–248.

Petti, V. L., Voelker, S. L., Shore, D. L., & Hayman-Abello, S. E. (2003). Perception of nonverbal emotion cues by children with nonverbal learning disabilities. *Journal of Developmental and Physical Disabilities*, *15*(1), 23–36.

Piaget, J. (1972). Development and learning. *Readings on the Development of Children*, 25–33.

Rigoni, F., Cornoldi, C., & Alcetti, A. (1997). Difficoltà nella comprensione e rappresentazione di descrizioni visuospaziali in bambini con disturbi non-verbali dell'apprendimento. *Psicologia Clinica dello Sviluppo*, *1*(2), 189–218.

Roman, M. A. (1998). The syndrome of nonverbal learning disabilities: Clinical description and applied aspects. *Current Issues in Education*, *1*(1), 1–21.

Rourke, B. P. (1989). *Nonverbal learning disabilities: The syndrome and the model.* Guilford Press.

Rourke, B. P. (2000). *Conference on nonverbal learning disabilities*, Speech delivered in New Haven, CT.

Rourke, B. P. (Ed.). (1995). *Syndrome of nonverbal learning disabilities: Neurodevelopmental manifestations.* Guilford Press.

Rourke, B. P., & Tsatsanis, K. D. (2000). Nonverbal learning disabilities and Asperger syndrome. *Asperger Syndrome*, 231–253.

Rourke, B. P., Young, G. C., & Leenaars, A. A. (1989). A childhood learning disability that predisposes those afflicted to adolescent and adult depression and suicide risk. *Journal of Learning Disabilities*, 22(3), 169–175.

Ryburn, B., Anderson, V., & Wales, R. (2009). Asperger syndrome: How does it relate to non-verbal learning disability? *Journal of Neuropsychology*, *3*(1), 107–123.

Schmidt, S., Tinti, C., Fantino, M., Mammarella, I. C., & Cornoldi, C. (2013). Spatial representations in blind people: The role of strategies and mobility skills. *Acta Psychologica*, *142*(1), 43–50.

Semrud-Clikeman, M. (2007). Social competence in children with nonverbal learning disabilities. *Social competence in children* (pp. 91–106). Boston, MA: Springer.

Semrud-Clikeman, M., & Fine, J. (2011). Presence of cysts on magnetic resonance images (MRIs) in children with Asperger disorder and nonverbal learning disabilities. *Journal of Child Neurology*, *26*(4), 471–475.

Semrud-Clikeman, M., & Glass, K. (2008). Comprehension of humor in children with nonverbal learning disabilities, reading disabilities, and without learning disabilities. *Annals of Dyslexia*, *58*(2), 163–180.

Semrud-Clikeman, M., & Hynd, G. W. (1990). Right hemisphere dysfunction in nonverbal learning disabilities: Social, academic, and adaptive functioning in adults and children. *Psychological Bulletin*, *107*(2), 196.

Semrud-Clikeman, M., Fine, J. G., & Bledsoe, J. (2014). Comparison among children with children with autism spectrum disorder, nonverbal learning disorder and typically developing children on measures of executive functioning. *Journal of Autism and Developmental Disorders*, *44*(2), 331–342.

Semrud-Clikeman, M., Fine, J. G., Bledsoe, J., & Zhu, D. C. (2013). Magnetic resonance imaging volumetric findings in children with Asperger syndrome, nonverbal learning disability, or healthy controls. *Journal of Clinical and Experimental Neuropsychology*, *35*(5), 540–550.

Semrud-Clikeman, M., Walkowiak, J., Wilkinson, A., & Christopher, G. (2010). Neuropsychological differences among children with Asperger syndrome, nonverbal learning disabilities, attention deficit disorder, and controls. *Developmental Neuropsychology*, *35*(5), 582–600.

Simic, N., Khan, S., & Rovet, J. (2013). Visuospatial, visuoperceptual, and visuoconstructive abilities in congenital hypothyroidism. *Journal of the International Neuropsychological Society: JINS*, *19*(10), 1119.

Somale, A., Kondekar, S., Rathi, S., & Iyer, N. (2016). Neurodevelopmental comorbidity profile in specific learning disorders. *International Journal of Contemporary Pediatrics*, *3*(2), 355–361.

Spreen, O. (2011). Nonverbal learning disabilities: A critical review. *Child Neuropsychology*, *17*(5), 418–443.

Staikova, E., Gomes, H., Tartter, V., McCabe, A., & Halperin, J. M. (2013). Pragmatic deficits and social impairment in children with ADHD. *Journal of Child Psychology and Psychiatry*, *54*(12), 1275–1283.

Tager-Flusberg, H. (1999). A psychological approach to understanding the social and language impairments in autism. *International Review of Psychiatry*, *11*(4), 325–334.

Tanguay, P. (2001). *Nonverbal learning disabilities at school: Educating students with NLD, Asperger syndrome and related conditions*. Jessica Kingsley Publishers.

Telzrow, C. F., & Bonar, A. M. (2002). Responding to students with nonverbal learning disabilities. *Teaching Exceptional Children*, *34*(6), 8–13.

Thomas, M. A., & Ollendick, T. H. (2008). A conceptual review of the comorbidity of attention-deficit/hyperactivity disorder and anxiety: Implications for future research and practice. *Child Psychology Review*, *28*, 1266–1280.

Thompson, S. (1997). *The source [R] for nonverbal learning disorders.* East Moline, IL: LinguiSystems, Inc.

Thompson, S. J., Auslander, W. F., & White, N. H. (2001). Comparison of single-mother and two-parent families on metabolic control of children with diabetes. *Diabetes Care*, *24*(2), 234–238.

Tranel, D., Hall, L. E., Olson, S., & Tranel, N. N. (1987). Evidence for a right-hemisphere developmental learning disability. *Developmental Neuropsychology*, *3*(2), 113–127.

Tsai, C. L., Wilson, P. H., & Wu, S. K. (2008). Role of visual–perceptual skills (non-motor) in children with developmental coordination disorder. *Human Movement Science*, *27*(4), 649–664.

Tsatsanis, K. D., & Rourke, B. P. (2003). Syndrome of nonverbal learning disabilities: Effects on learning. *Therapist's guide to learning and attention disorders*, 109–145.

Tsur, V. G., Shalev, R. S., Manor, O., & Amir, N. (1995). Developmental right-hemisphere syndrome: Clinical spectrum of the nonverbal learning disability. *Journal of Learning Disabilities*, *28*(2), 80–86.

Tuley, K., & Bell, N. (1997). *On cloud nine*. San Luis Obispo, CA.

Tunali, B., & Power, T. G. (1993). Creating satisfaction: A psychological perspective on stress and coping in families of handicapped children. *Journal of Child Psychology and Psychiatry*, *34*(6), 945–957.

Uttal, D. H., Miller, D. I., & Newcombe, N. S. (2013). Exploring and enhancing spatial thinking: Links to achievement in science, technology, engineering, and mathematics? *Current Directions in Psychological Science*, *22*(5), 367–373.

Van Luit, J. E. H., & Van de Rijt, B. A. M. (2009). *Utrechtse getalbegrip toets — revised.* [Early Numeracy Test–Revised]. Doetinchem, Netherlands: Graviant.

Vance, A., Silk, T. J., Casey, M., Rinehart, N. J., Bradshaw, J. L., Bellgrove, M. A., & Cunnington, R. (2007). Right parietal dysfunction in children with attention deficit hyperactivity disorder, combined type: A functional MRI study. *Molecular Psychiatry*, *12*(9), 826–832.

Venneri, A., Cornoldi, C., & Garuti, M. (2003). Arithmetic difficulties in children with visuospatial learning disability (VLD). *Child Neuropsychology*, *9*(3), 175–183.

Volkmar, F. R., & Klin, A. (2000). Diagnostic issues in Asperger syndrome. *Asperger Syndrome*, *27*, 25–71.

Wai, J., Lubinski, D., & Benbow, C. P. (2009). Spatial ability for STEM domains: Aligning over 50 years of cumulative psychological knowledge solidifies its importance. *Journal of Educational Psychology*, *101*(4), 817.

Webster-Stratton, C. (1990). Stress: A potential disruptor of parent perceptions and family interactions. *Journal of Clinical Child Psychology*, *19*(4), 302–312.

Weintraub, S., & Mesulam, M. M. (1983). Developmental learning disabilities of the right hemisphere: Emotional, interpersonal, and cognitive components. *Archives of Neurology*, *40*(8), 463–468.

Whitney, R. V. (2002). *Bridging the gap: Raising a child with nonverbal learning disorder*. Penguin.

Wilkinson-Smith, A., & Semrud-Clikeman, M. (2014). Are fine-motor impairments a defining feature of nonverbal learning disabilities in children? *Applied Neuropsychology: Child*, *3*(1), 52–59.

Willcutt, E. G., Doyle, A. E., Nigg, J. T., Faraone, S. V., & Pennington, B. F. (2005). Validity of the executive function theory of attention-deficit/hyperactivity disorder: A meta-analytic review. *Biological Psychiatry*, *57*(11), 1336–1346.

Williams, D. L., Goldstein, G., Kojkowski, N., & Minshew, N. J. (2008). Do individuals with high functioning autism have the IQ profile associated with nonverbal learning disability? *Research in Autism Spectrum Disorders*, *2*(2), 353–361.

Wilson, P. H., Maruff, P., Butson, M., Williams, J., Lum, J., & Thomas, P. R. (2004). Internal representation of movement in children with developmental coordination disorder: A mental rotation task. *Developmental Medicine & Child Neurology*, *46*(11), 754–759.

Worling, D. E., Humphries, T., & Tannock, R. (1999). Spatial and emotional aspects of language inferencing in nonverbal learning disabilities. *Brain and Language*, *70*(2), 220–239.

Zimmer, H. D., Speiser, H. R., & Seidler, B. (2003). Spatio-temporal working-memory and short-term object-location tasks use different memory mechanisms. *Acta Psychologica*, *114*(1), 41–65.

Index